Reflex Seizures and Related Epileptic Syndromes

C.P. Panayiotopoulos

Reflex Seizures and Related Epileptic Syndromes

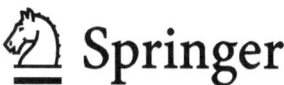 Springer

Author
C.P. Panayiotopoulos M.D., Ph.D., F.R.C.P.
Department of Clinical Neurophysiology and Epilepsies
St Thomas' Hospital
London
United Kingdom

ISBN 978-1-4471-4041-2   ISBN 978-1-4471-4042-9   (eBook)
DOI 10.1007/978-1-4471-4042-9
Springer Dordrecht Heidelberg New York London

Library of Congress Control Number: 2012941298

Printed on acid-free paper

Springer is part of Springer Science+Business Media (www.springer.com)

Preface

Of patients with epilepsy, 4–7% have reflex seizures alone or together with spontaneous seizures.

Reflex epileptic seizures denote epileptic seizures that are consistently elicited by a specific 'precipitating' stimulus. The term 'precipitating stimulus' should be differentiated from 'facilitating stimulus'. In some patients for example EEG discharges or seizures may increase during intermittent photic stimulation (IPS) (facilitating stimulus), but are not consistently evoked by IPS (as would be expected with precipitating stimuli).

The precipitating stimulus evoking an epileptic seizure is specific for a given patient and may be extrinsic, intrinsic or both. Extrinsic stimuli are (a) simple, such as flashes of light, elimination of visual fixation and tactile stimuli and (b) complex, such as reading or music. Intrinsic stimuli are elementary, such as movements, or elaborate, such as those involving higher brain function, emotions and cognition (thinking, calculating, music or decision-making). Intermittent photic stimulation is the most common stimulus triggering epileptic seizures.

Reflex seizures may be (a) generalised, such as absences, myoclonic jerks or generalised tonic clonic seizures or (b) focal, such as visual, motor or sensory.

The role of the EEG is fundamental in establishing the precipitating stimulus in reflex epilepsies, because it allows subclinical EEG reflex abnormalities, or minor clinical ictal events, to be reproduced on demand by application of the appropriate stimulus without risk to the patient. However, there are cases in which the stimulus–seizure relationship is difficult to document, as in video game-induced seizures.

Management is syndrome related. Antiepileptic drugs may not be needed in patients with reflex seizures only. Avoidance of precipitating stimulus may be adequate.

This concise booklet provides a physician-friendly modern review of all types of reflex seizures and related reflex epilepsy syndromes that I have studied from the early days of my medical career (Ph.D. on photosensitive epilepsy) and continue to date (fixation-off sensitivity, Jeavons syndrome, reading epilepsy). Prevalence, clinical features, EEG manifestations, pathophysiology and treatment are meaningfully described. Key points of practical clinical significance are emphasised. The aim is to assist health care professionals in optimising the diagnosis and management of patients with reflex seizures.

2012 March Oxford   C.P. Panayiotopoulos, M.D., Ph.D., F.R.C.P.

Contents

Introduction xiii

Part I   Visually Induced Seizures and Related Epilepsies

Chapter 1:
Photosensitivity, Epileptic Seizures and Epileptic Syndromes 3
  Clarifications on Classification
  Demographic Data
  Clinical Manifestations
    Generalised Seizures
    Focal Seizures
    Precipitating Factors
    Self-induced Photic Reflex Seizures
  Aetiology
  Diagnostic Procedures
  Prognosis
  Management
    Avoidance or Prevention of the Provocative Stimulus May Be the Only Treatment
  AED Treatment

Chapter 2:
Idiopathic Photosensitive Occipital Lobe Epilepsy 15
  Clarifications on Classification
  Demographic Data
  Clinical Manifestations
    Precipitating Factors
  Diagnostic Procedures
    Electroencephalography
  Aetiology
  Differential Diagnosis
  Prognosis
  Management

Chapter 3:
Jeavons Syndrome 21
  Considerations on Classification
  Demographic Data
  Clinical Manifestations
    Precipitating Factors
    Self-induction in Jeavons Syndrome
  Aetiology
    Pathophysiology

Diagnostic Procedures
  Electroencephalography
Differential Diagnosis
Prognosis
Management

Chapter 4:
Pattern-Sensitive Epilepsy 27
Demographic Data
Clinical Manifestations
  Environmental Stimuli
Aetiology
  Pathophysiology
Diagnostic Procedures
Prognosis
Management

Chapter 5:
Fixation-off Sensitivity 31
Clinical and EEG Correlations in Patients with FOS
  Pathophysiology
Scotosensitive Epilepsy
Techniques for Documenting FOS

Part II   Complex Reflex Epilepsies

Chapter 6:
Seizures Induced by Thinking and Praxis 37

Chapter 7:
Primary (Idiopathic) Reading Epilepsy 39
Clarifications on Classification
Demographic Data
Clinical Manifestations
  Precipitating Factors
Aetiology
  Pathophysiology
Diagnostic Procedures
  Electroencephalography
Prognosis
Management

Chapter 8:
Startle Seizures 43
Clarifications on Classification
Demographic Data
Clinical Manifestations
Aetiology
Diagnostic Procedures
  Electroencephalography

Differential Diagnosis
Prognosis
Management

Chapter 9:
Hot Water Epilepsy 47
  Clarifications on Classification
  Demographic Data
  Clinical Manifestations
  Aetiology
    Pathophysiology
  Diagnostic Procedures
    Electroencephalography
  Differential Diagnosis
  Prognosis
  Management

References 51

Index 59

Abbreviations

AED	Anti-epileptic drug
EEG	Electroencephalogram
FDA	US Food & Drug Administration
fMRI	Functional magnetic resonance imaging
FOS	Fixation-off sensitivity
GSWD	Generalised spike–wave discharges
GTCS	Generalised tonic–clonic seizure
ICOE-G	Idiopathic childhood occipital epilepsy of Gastaut
IGE	Idiopathic generalised epilepsy
ILAE	International League Against Epilepsy
IPOE	Idiopathic photosensitive occipital lobe epilepsy
IPS	Intermittent photic stimulation
JME	Juvenile myoclonic epilepsy
MEG	Magnetoencephalography
MRI	Magnetic resonance imaging
OPS	Occipital seizures precipitated by photic stimuli
PET	Positron emission tomography
PPR	Photoparoxysmal response
VER	Visual evoked response

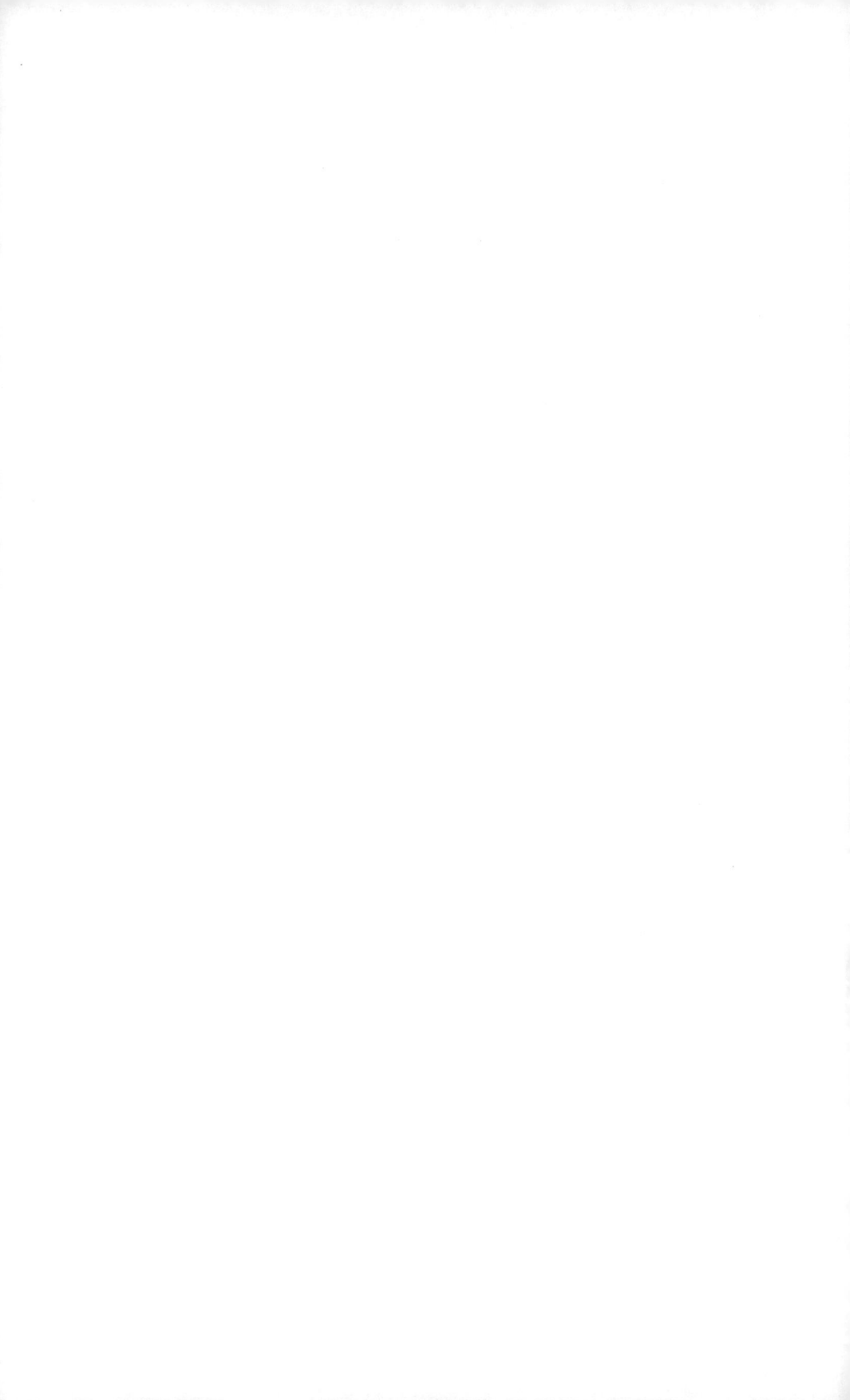

Introduction

Epileptic seizures can arise in a 'spontaneous' unpredictable fashion with no detectable precipitating factors, or they can be provoked by certain recognisable stimuli.

Factors and stimuli that contribute towards the initiation of a seizure are provided by the individual's internal and external environment. Hormones, electrolytes, state of consciousness and body temperature are examples of internal factors that alter the epileptogenic threshold. External factors may be sensory, electrical or biochemical. A complex interaction between external and internal factors may explain why the effectiveness of a well-defined seizure-precipitating stimulus may vary and why a patient may experience both 'spontaneous' and 'reflex' seizures.

Reflex seizures have a 4–7% prevalence among patients with epilepsies. Their aetiology may be idiopathic, symptomatic or cryptogenic (probably symptomatic).

Clarifications on Classification

Reflex or stimulus-sensitive, or triggered or sensory evoked, epileptic seizures are synonyms denoting epileptic seizures that are consistently elicited by a specific stimulus.[1-4] 'Reflex' is the preferred name in the new ILAE diagnostic scheme[5] and report[6] (Table 1).

The ILAE report classifies reflex epilepsies under an unspecified category of 'special epilepsy conditions'.[6] The list of special epilepsy conditions is:

- Symptomatic focal epilepsies not otherwise specified
- Epilepsy with generalised tonic–clonic seizures (GTCSs) only
- Reflex epilepsies
- Febrile seizures plus (FS+)
- Familial focal epilepsy with variable foci

Reflex epilepsies: Although idiopathic photosensitive occipital lobe epilepsy, primary reading epilepsy and hot water epilepsy in infants are syndromes, it is unclear whether other reflex epilepsies constitute unique syndromes.[6]

Precipitating stimuli for reflex seizures
Visual stimuli
   Flickering light – colour to be specified when possible
   Patterns
   Other visual stimuli
Thinking
Music
Eating
Praxis
Somatosensory
Proprioceptive
Reading
Hot water
Startle
Reflex seizures
Reflex seizures in generalised epilepsy syndromes
Reflex seizures in focal epilepsy syndromes
Reflex epilepsies[a]
Idiopathic photosensitive occipital lobe epilepsy (2)
Other visual-sensitive epilepsies
Primary reading epilepsy (3)
Startle epilepsy[b]
Hot water epilepsy in infants (2)[c]
Conditions with epileptic seizures that do not require a diagnosis of epilepsy
Reflex seizures

Modified with permission from Engel[5,6]

[a]Numbers in parenthesis indicate rating of confidence regarding the certainty with which the ILAE Core Group believed each syndrome represented a unique diagnostic entity (3 being the most clearly and reproducibly defined)

[b]The new ILAE report[6] rightly no longer considers startle epilepsy to be an epilepsy syndrome

[c]Hot water epilepsy in infants has been newly considered an epileptic syndrome by the ILAE[6]

Table 1 Precipitating stimuli and reflex seizures and syndromes listed in the ILAE classification scheme[5,6]

Definitions

Reflex seizures are:

Objectively and consistently demonstrated to be evoked by a specific afferent stimulus or by activity of the patient. Afferent stimuli can be elementary, i.e. unstructured (light flashes, startle, a monotone), or elaborate, i.e. structured. Activity may be *elementary*, e.g. motor (a movement), or *elaborate*, e.g. cognitive function (reading, chess playing), or both (reading aloud).[7]

Reflex epilepsy syndrome is:

A syndrome in which *all* epileptic seizures are precipitated by sensory stimuli. Reflex seizures that occur in focal and generalized epilepsy syndromes that are also associated with spontaneous seizures are listed as seizure types. Isolated reflex seizures can also occur in situations that do not necessarily require a diagnosis of epilepsy. Seizures precipitated by other special circumstances, such as fever or alcohol withdrawal, are not reflex seizures.[5]

Reflex epilepsies are determined by the specific precipitating stimulus and the clinico-EEG response.[1,2,8]

The Precipitating Stimulus

The stimulus evoking an epileptic seizure is specific for a given patient and may be extrinsic, intrinsic or both.

Extrinsic stimuli are:

- Simple, such as flashes of light, elimination of visual fixation and tactile stimuli
- Complex, such as reading or music

The latency from the stimulus onset to the clinical or EEG response is typically short (1–3 s) with simple stimuli or long (usually many minutes) with complex stimuli.

Intrinsic stimuli are:

- Elementary, such as movements
- Elaborate, such as those involving higher brain function, emotions and cognition (thinking, calculating, music or decision-making).

Author's Note

In the ILAE definition of reflex epilepsy syndromes, 'all seizures are precipitated by sensory stimuli' may be too restrictive. Most patients also suffer from spontaneous seizures. Should 'all' be replaced by 'all or nearly all'?

The term 'precipitating stimulus' should be differentiated from 'facilitating stimulus'. In certain patients with idiopathic generalised epilepsy (IGE), for example, EEG discharges or seizures may increase during intermittent photic stimulation (IPS; facilitating stimulus) but these are not consistently evoked by IPS (as would be expected with precipitating stimuli).

The Response to the Stimulus

The response to the stimulus consists of clinical and EEG manifestations, alone or in combination. EEG activation may be electrographic (subclinical) only, i.e. without overt clinical manifestations. Conversely, ictal clinical manifestations may be triggered without conspicuous surface EEG changes.

Clinical Types of Reflex Seizure

Reflex seizures may be:

- Generalised, such as absences, myoclonic jerks or GTCSs
- Focal, such as visual, motor or sensory

Reflex generalised seizures occur either independently or within the broad framework of certain epileptic syndromes. The same patient, in response to the same specific stimulus, may have absences, myoclonic jerks and GTCSs alone, or in various combinations. Usually, absences and myoclonic jerks precede the occurrence of GTCSs. Patients may have reflex and spontaneous seizures.

Myoclonic jerks are by far the most common, and manifest in the limbs and trunk or regionally, such as in the eyelids (eyelid myoclonia with absences).

GTCSs may occur from the start, constituting the first clinical response, or more commonly they follow a cluster of absences or myoclonic jerks. Secondarily GTCSs from focal, simple or complex seizures are much less common than primarily GTCSs.

Absence seizures are common, constituting the response to a variety of specific stimuli, such as photic, pattern, fixation-off, proprioceptive, cognitive, emotional or linguistic stimuli.[9] It is recognised that absences are also common in self-induction.

Focal seizures are exclusively seen in certain types of reflex focal or lobular epilepsy, such as visual seizures of photosensitive occipital lobe epilepsy or complex focal temporal lobe seizures of musicogenic epilepsy.

Reflex-Electroclinical Events and the Role of the EEG

The electroclinical events may be strictly limited to the stimulus-related receptive brain region only (such as photically induced EEG occipital spikes), spread to other cortical areas (such as in photosensitive focal seizures that propagate in extraoccipital areas) or become generalised (e.g. in the photoparoxysmal responses [PPRs] of an IGE). Furthermore, the electroclinical response to a specific stimulus may correspond to activation of regions other than those of the relevant receptive area, such as in primary reading epilepsy, which manifests with jaw myoclonic jerks. Conversely, reading may elicit electroclinical events strictly confined to the brain regions subserving reading, such as alexia, associated with focal ictal EEG paroxysms. There is great variability in the interindividual responses to the same stimulus.

The role of the EEG is fundamental in establishing the precipitating stimulus in reflex epilepsies, because it allows subclinical EEG reflex abnormalities, or minor clinical ictal events, to be reproduced on demand by application of the appropriate stimulus without risk to the patient. However, there are cases in which the stimulus–seizure relationship is difficult to document, as in video game-induced seizures. Only 70% of these patients have EEG confirmation of photosensitivity with PPRs to IPS, and in the other 30% seizures may be due to a single or a variety of other precipitating or facilitating stimuli. Sleep deprivation, mental concentration, fatigue, excitement, borderline threshold to photosensitivity, fixation-off sensitivity (FOS), proprioceptive stimuli (praxis), or more complex visual or auditory stimuli, alone or in combination, are all possibilities that are difficult to document objectively with an EEG.[10–12] There are also epileptic syndromes in which EEG 'epileptogenic activity' is consistently elicited by a specific stimulus with no apparent clinical relevance. This is exemplified by certain cases of benign focal childhood seizures in which somatosensory (tapping) or visual (elimination of fixation and central vision) stimuli consistently elicit spike activity, although these children appear to have 'unprovoked' seizures that mainly occur during sleep.[12]

Table 2 provides an analytical list of reflex seizures, related reflex epileptic syndromes and their precipitating stimuli. Some of these, such as photosensitivity, are well known and common, but others are extremely rare in humans, although they may be common in animals, such as audiogenic seizures.

I. Simple somatosensory stimuli

1. Exteroceptive somatosensory stimuli
   (a) Tapping epilepsy and benign childhood epilepsy with somatosensory evoked spikes[17–20]
   (b) Sensory (tactile) evoked idiopathic myoclonic seizures in infancy[21]
   (c) Toothbrushing epilepsy[22,23]
2. Complex exteroceptive somatosensory stimuli
   (a) Hot water epilepsy[24]
3. Simple proprioceptive somatosensory stimuli
   (a) Seizures induced by movements[25]
   (b) Seizures induced by eye closure and/or eye movements[26]
   (c) Paroxysmal kinesigenic choreoathetosis[27]
   (d) Seizures induced by micturition[28,29]
4. Complex proprioceptive stimuli
   (a) Eating epilepsy[30,31]

II. Visual stimuli

1. Simple visual stimuli
   (a) Photosensitive epilepsies (including self-induced photosensitive epilepsy)[13,16,32]
   (b) Pattern-sensitive epilepsies[13,33,34] (including self-induced pattern-sensitive epilepsy)[35]
   (c) Fixation-off sensitive epilepsies[36]
   (d) Scotogenic epilepsy[36]
2. Complex visual stimuli and language processing (language-induced seizures)
   (a) Reading epilepsy[37–41]
   (b) Graphogenic epilepsy[42,43]

III. Auditory, vestibular, olfactory and gustatory stimuli[25,44]

(a) Seizures induced by pure sounds or words[25]
(b) Audiogenic seizures[45]
(c) Musicogenic epilepsy (and singing epilepsy)[46,47]
(d) Telephone-induced seizures[48]
(e) Olfactorhinencephalic epilepsy[1]
(f) Eating epilepsy triggered by tastes[31]
(g) Seizures triggered by vestibular and auditory stimuli[25]

IV. Seizures induced by high-level processes (cognitive, emotional, decision-making tasks and other complex stimuli)[44,49]

(a) Thinking (noogenic) epilepsy[49–51]
(b) Praxis-induced seizures[49,52]
(c) Emotional epilepsies[53–55]
(d) Startle epilepsy[56]

Modified with permission from Panayiotopoulos[8]
For further details, see the literature[1–3]

Table 2 Reflex seizures, related reflex syndromes and the precipitating stimuli

In this book, common and principal forms of simple and complex reflex seizures and epilepsies are reviewed with particular emphasis on the syndromes listed in the new ILAE diagnostic scheme.[5] Classic references or reviews are cited for the remainder.

Part I

Visually Induced Seizures and Related Epilepsies[1,2,8,13–16]

Seizures triggered by visual stimuli are the most common type of reflex seizure. Visual seizures are triggered by the physical characteristics of the visual stimuli and not by their cognitive effects. Photosensitivity and pattern sensitivity are the two main categories (with frequent overlap) of simple reflex epilepsies, with a short (typically within seconds) time period between stimulus and response. Photosensitivity and pattern sensitivity are genetically determined.

Video-EEG samples of many patients with photically induced seizures or other reflex epileptic seizures can be seen in the CD companion of references[57–60].

Photosensitivity, Epileptic Seizures and Epileptic Syndromes

Photosensitivity, an abnormal reflex EEG paroxysmal activation by photic stimulation (PPR), is a genetically determined trait. Reflex photic EEG activation may be asymptomatic throughout life or manifest with clinical epileptic seizures. 'Photosensitive epilepsy' is a broad term comprising numerous heterogeneous disorders in which seizures are triggered by light. It is not an epilepsy syndrome. Some recognised epileptic syndromes show a high incidence of clinically manifested epileptic seizures and, more frequently, PPRs without clinical seizures.

Clarifications on Classification

Photosensitivity epilepsy was classified among the generalised epilepsies by the ILAE Commission.[4] This is for the following reasons:

- PPRs were considered to be primarily generalised,[1,13,61,62] although the initial occipital onset of the discharge was well reported[63,64] and recently appreciated.[3,13,65] The evidence is that photosensitivity in humans is mainly generated in the occipital lobes and therefore it is a regional (occipital lobar) epilepsy.
- A quarter of patients with spontaneous seizures and EEG photosensitivity belong to a variety of epileptic syndromes of IGE, such as juvenile myoclonic epilepsy (JME).[8,66] A high prevalence of photosensitivity is also found in certain forms of symptomatic generalised epilepsies, such as Dravet syndrome (70%), and Unverricht disease.

Occipital photosensitivity only recently came into prominence, although it has been well known from the time of Gowers (1881).[67] This was overshadowed by the prevailing view that photosensitive epilepsies are mainly generalised. Indeed, with the application of IPS as a provocation method in EEG, it was discovered that most photosensitivity patients had generalised discharges and suffered mainly from IGEs.[68,69] That occipital spikes often preceded generalised discharges[63,64,70] was ignored. Reports of photically induced occipital seizures with or without secondary generalisation were scarce. The traditional view that occipital seizures precipitated by photic stimuli (OPSs) are rare contrasts with recent findings.[71–73] In one report alone,[74] 45 of 95 patients had occipital seizures precipitated by visual stimuli. There are two recommended, extensive reviews on OPSs.[12,75]

C.P. Panayiotopoulos, *Reflex Seizures and Related Epileptic Syndromes*,
DOI 10.1007/978-1-4471-4042-9_1, © Springer-Verlag London 2012

Demographic Data[13,76,77]

The onset of photic reflex seizures can occur at any age, but they mainly start at 7–19 years with a peak at 12 or 13 years. Two-thirds are women.[13,76] PPRs occur in 1/4000 of the population and 5% of patients with epileptic seizures.[78,79] The overall annual incidence of cases with a newly presenting seizure and unequivocal photosensitivity in the UK is 1.1/100,000 (2% of all new cases with epileptic seizures). When restricted to the age range of 7–19 years, the annual incidence rises to 5.7/100,000 (10% of all new cases with epileptic seizures in this age group).[78,79] In healthy males aged between 17 and 25 years, EEG photosensitivity is very low (0.35%).[78–80]

Clinical Manifestations

These vary considerably depending on syndrome and severity of photosensitivity. Of seizure patients with PPRs:

- 42% have only photically induced reflex seizures without spontaneous seizures (*pure photosensitive epilepsy*)
- 40% have spontaneous and reflex photosensitive seizures
- The remaining 18% have spontaneous seizures only.

Some recognised syndromes of IGE, such as JME, show a high incidence of clinical, but, more often, EEG photosensitivity.

> *Generalised seizures are much more common than occipital ones; any other focal seizures from other brain regions are exceptional at the start.*

Generalised Seizures

Myoclonic jerks, absences and GTCSs can occur, in this order by prevalence, in photosensitive patients. Some patients may have only one type, but most have any combination, particularly myoclonic jerks and GTCSs. That myoclonic jerks are by far the most common may appear contradictory to the ordinarily stated view that GTCSs prevail.[13] Thus, GTCSs are reported far more frequently (55–84%) than absences (6–20%), focal seizures (2.5%) and myoclonic jerks (2–8%). This prevalence is based on clinical historical evidence, which is likely to over-exaggerate GTCSs in relation to minor seizure events, even though they predominate. In 75% of patients with photosensitivity, PPRs are associated with ictal impairment of consciousness or motor symptoms (opening of the eyes, eyelid or other myoclonic jerks), although these are not reported by a third of patients.[81,82] In my personal experience with video-EEG, PPRs are commonly associated with eyelid manifestations (a blink, fluttering, flickering, myoclonia) and less often with jerks of the head, eyes, body or limbs. Absences followed in prevalence and only one patient had an accidental GTCS. Patients are often unaware of minor seizures, although some of these may be sufficiently obvious and marked. These facts have been illustrated on many occasions in my book 83a (see, for example, Figs. 1.1 and 1.2).

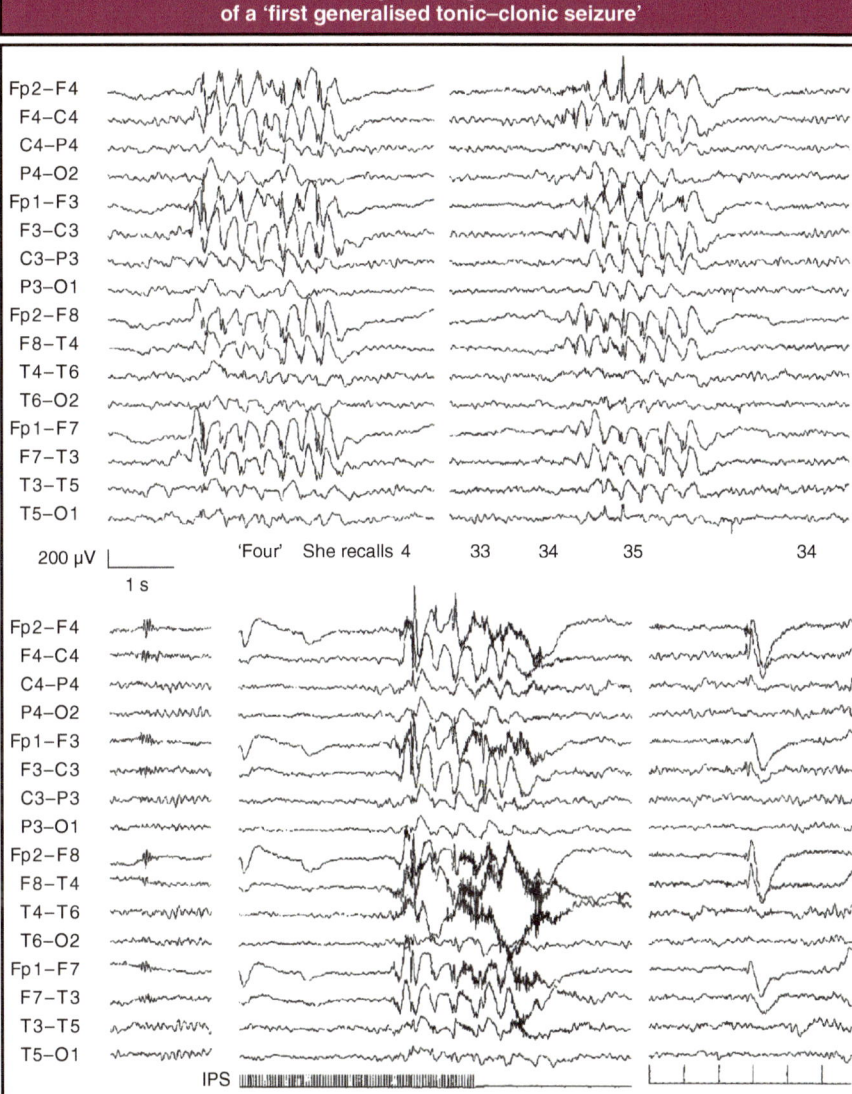

Fig. 1.1 This girl had her first GTCS in the morning on her way to school for examinations. She suddenly became vague and nearly simultaneously fell on the ground with generalised convulsions. On questioning by the EEG technologist, it was revealed that 1 year before the GTCS she had mild jerks of the fingers in the morning interpreted as clumsiness. The EEG had generalised discharges of 3–4 Hz spike/multispike and slow wave. The girl recalled the number shouted to her during the discharge. However, breath counting during hyperventilation was disturbed during a similar discharge (annotated numbers). In addition, there were photoparoxysmal discharges. Brief frontal asymmetrical bursts of polyspikes or spike and slow wave could be erroneously interpreted as 'frontal lobe epilepsy with secondary bilateral synchrony'. On clinical and EEG grounds the diagnosis of JME was established and appropriate treatment was initiated because she had many more seizures (myoclonic jerks) prior and in addition to the single GTCS

Sample from a video-EEG of a woman, aged 28 years, who had suffered from JME since the age of 9 years

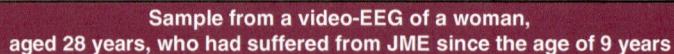

Treatment stopped at age18 years despite myoclonic jerks and brief absences – first GTCS at age 28
a
first
Fp2–F4
F4–C4
C4–P4
P4–O2
Fp1–F3
F3–C3
C3–P3
P3–O1
Counting interrupted – eyelid jerk with each spike/polyspike 300 µV
1 s
b
Fp2–F4
F4–C4
C4–P4
P4–O2
Fp1–F3
F3–C3
C3–P3
P3–O1
IPS
Eyelid jerks with each spike/polyspike 300 µV
1 s
c
Fp1–F3
100 µV
1 s

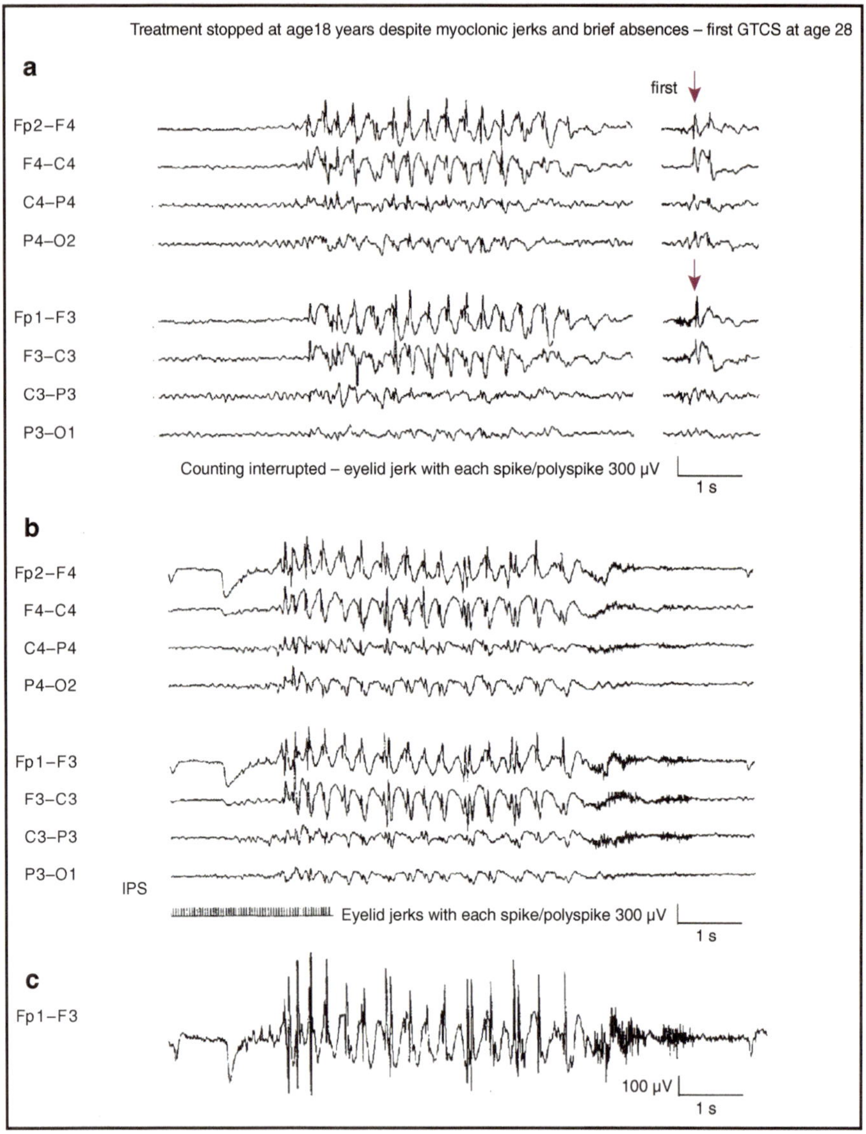

Fig. 1.2 This woman was referred for a routine EEG because she had experienced 'probable IGE-absences from age 9 until age 18 years. Myoclonus as a teenager when sleep deprived. Recently suffered her first ever GTCS following sleep deprivation. No absence or myoclonus for 10 years. Treatment with valproate was withdrawn at age 18 years.' The video-EEG documented that she still had brief absences, which manifest with mild impairment of cognition and eyelid jerks. These were spontaneous, or induced by (**a**) hyperventilation and (**b**) intermittent photic stimulation. Note the polyspike–wave of the discharges and the irregular intradischarge frequency (**c**). Also note the bifrontal spike-slow wave discharges (**a**, *red arrows*)

Focal Seizures

Photically induced occipital seizures are much more frequent than was origi-
nally appreciated before the use of IPS in EEG testing. These may occur alone
or progress to symptoms from other brain locations and GTCSs. See also
'Idiopathic photosensitive occipital lobe epilepsy'.

Extra-occipital focal seizures from the onset are exceptional.[83]

Useful Note

Subjective symptoms during PPRs

These are of doubtful significance; some are ictal phenomena but most are not.[14] Many people
cannot tolerate the light at all, but this is not evidence of epileptic photosensitivity.

Precipitating Factors

By definition all patients are sensitive to flickering lights. Many artificial or
natural light sources can provoke epileptic seizures. Video games, television,
visual display units of computers, stroboscopic lights in discotheques and
natural flickering light are common triggers, in that order of prevalence.

Video game-induced seizures can occur not only with games using an
interlaced video monitor (television) but also with small hand-held liquid
crystal displays and non-interlaced 70 Hz arcade games.[10,84] Most patients
(87%) are aged 7–19 years. There is a preponderance of boys, probably
because more boys play video games than girls. Two-thirds of patients are
photosensitive; for the other third there are other triggers such as sleep deprivation, fatigue, decision making, excitement or frustration, and praxis, which
may all operate alone or in combination.[11] A third of video game-induced
seizures are occipital seizures and these occur in patients with or without
photosensitivity.

Television epilepsy denotes seizures triggered by television and it is not a
syndrome. Television-induced seizures mainly affect children aged 10–12 years.
There is a twofold preponderance of girls. Seizures are more likely to occur
when the patient is watching a faulty (i.e. flickering) television set or is sitting
very near to the television screen. Myoclonic jerks often precede the GTCSs
and the history taken reveals that these may have occurred in the past without
GTCSs.

> *First she jerked a few times, head and hands, and then she had the
> convulsions. I thought she was electrocuted by an electric fault of
> the television.*

A substantial number of these patients also have spontaneous attacks. In
pure television epilepsy, one or a few overt television-induced seizures occur
without evidence of any other type of spontaneous seizure or seizures induced
by other means.

Ten percent of patients are 'drawn like a magnet' to the screen and when they have reached a certain nearness they have a GTCS.[13] This is called 'compulsive attraction'.

> *He was watching television and then suddenly, off he goes towards the set, eyes fixed in the picture, and he had the fit a few inches away from the screen.*
> *I do not know what happened. My eyes suddenly fixed to the picture, I could not move them away and then I passed out.*

Self-induced Photic Reflex Seizures[32,85–87]

Self-induction is a mode of seizure precipitation employed by mentally handicapped or normal photosensitive individuals. Its prevalence is debatable. Techniques include waving the outspread fingers in front of a bright light, viewing geometric patterns or slow eye closure. Absences and myoclonic jerks are the most common seizures in self-induction. Whether eyelid blinking or compulsive attraction to television or bright sun is mainly an attempt for self-induction or part of the seizure is disputed, although both may be true. In my opinion, in the majority of such cases these events are reflex seizure onsets.[85]

Aetiology

Photosensitivity is genetically determined. In particular, the genetic basis for PPRs has been well documented. Monozygotic twin studies have shown an almost 100% concordance. Family studies indicate a sibling risk between 20% and 50%, the latter when siblings are studied between 5 and 15 years of age with one of the parents also being affected. These indicate autosomal dominant inheritance with age-related reduced penetrance in PPR-positive patients who have seizures and in non-seizure individuals. However, PPRs also occur in a number of autosomal recessive diseases.[88] In one study of 32 clinically photosensitive mothers with 67 children, 13 children (20%) had PPRs and 4 also had clinical photosensitive seizures. Nine other EEG-examined children did not have PPRs.[89]

In recent studies of photosensitivity, linkage was found with chromosomes 7q32 and 16p13[90,91] or 6p21.2 and 13q31.3.[92] The gene encoding NEDD4-2, a ubiquitin protein ligase, has recently been implicated in some families with photosensitive generalised epilepsy.[93]

The role of exogenous factors is indicated by the example of two monozygotic twins with PPRs. Only one developed clinical photosensitive epilepsy after a period of weekly exposures to high-intensity light flashes.[94]

A European consortium on the genetic analysis of photosensitivity and visual-sensitive epilepsies is in progress.

Diagnostic Procedures

Properly applied IPS during EEG is the most important test.

IPS techniques vary significantly between publications and departments. I follow the recommendations made by Jeavons.[13] To be provocative, the IPS has to imply all potent physical characteristics of the stimulus (intensity, frequency, contrast) and combine flash with patterns, and central vision is mandatory (the patient should look at the centre of the stroboscope). IPS on eye closure should be tested.[13,95,96] Monocular stimulation is usually ineffective. Adding a quadrille pattern of small squares (2×2 mm) of fine black lines (0.33 mm) in the front of the stroboscope increases the possibility of obtaining PPRs.[97]

Warning

Prolonged photic stimulation that may expose the patient to a major convulsive seizure should be totally discouraged. There is nothing to learn or benefit from this practice. There are plenty of examples of individuals having an IPS-induced GTCS during an EEG that was performed for reasons other than epilepsy. To continue a train of photic stimulation after the appearance of EEG ictal discharges or ictal clinical manifestations is unacceptable.

The practical objective of IPS is to determine the following:
- Whether seizures (of any type) are aetiologically linked with environmental photic stimuli (television, video games and others); if PPRs occur, this confirms photosensitivity
- Whether PPRs are associated with ictal events; this requires video-EEG recording, otherwise minor events such as eyelid or limb jerks are likely to escape.

Useful Note

The duration of PPRs and their relationship to the IPS train

Emphasis is often given to whether PPRs outlast the stimulus train or whether they are self-limited, i.e. they stop before or with the end of the IPS.[95,96] The rationale is that PPRs that outlast the stimulus train may strengthen their association with epilepsy. This may be artificial because the duration of the discharge, as a rule, depends on the duration and strength of the IPS and the time that this is stopped after the onset of PPRs.

PPRs are broadly categorised as:[13,98]
- *Generalised spike/polyspike–waves:* They are of higher amplitude in the anterior regions, but onset – particularly if patterned IPS is employed – is often with occipital spikes. They are highly associated (90%) with clinical photosensitivity, particularly if they outlast the stimulus train (Fig. 1.3). Generalised PPRs often (60%) associate with clinical events such as jerks, impairment of cognition or subjective sensations, but their detection may require video-EEG.[98]

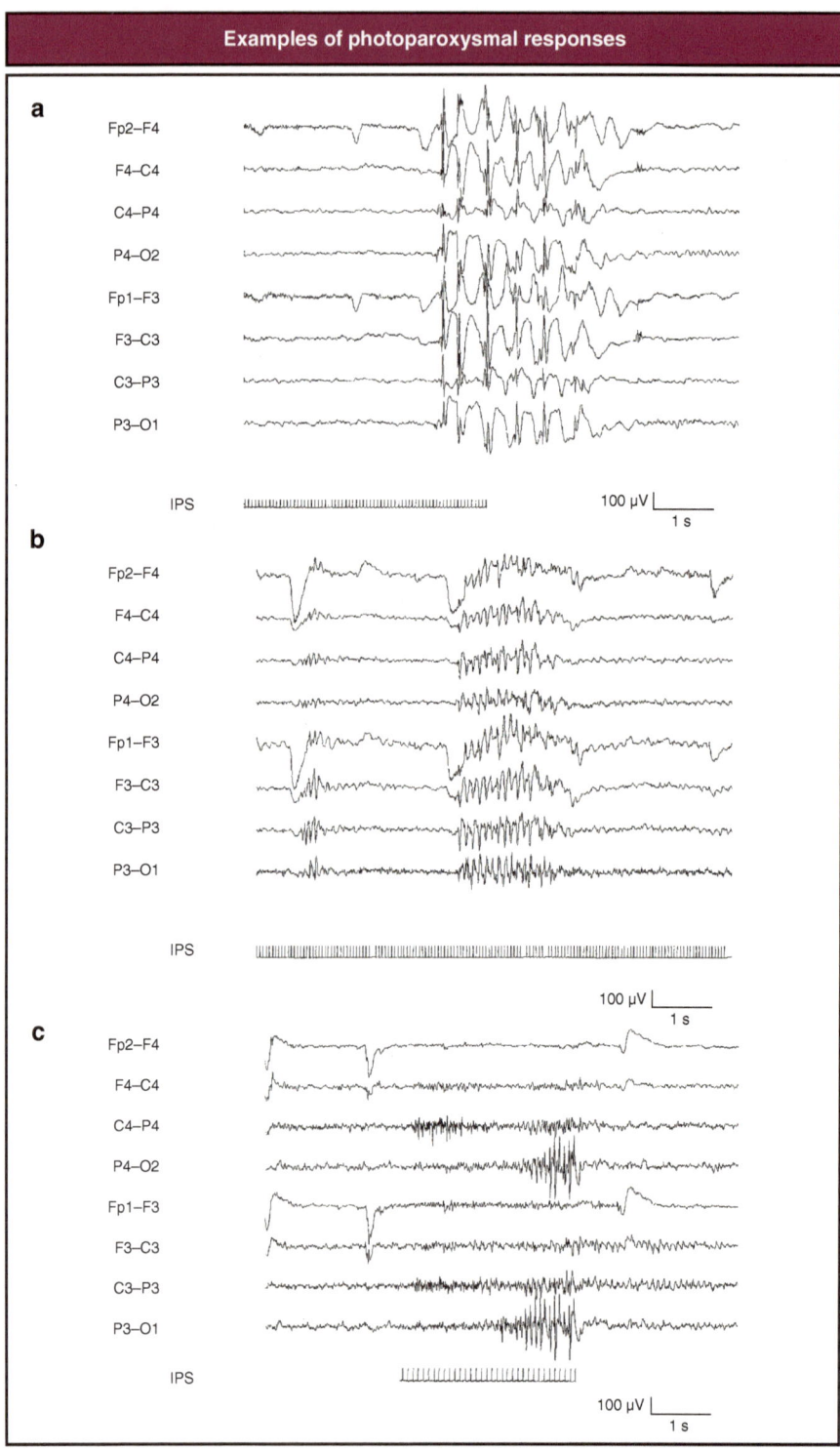

Examples of photoparoxysmal responses

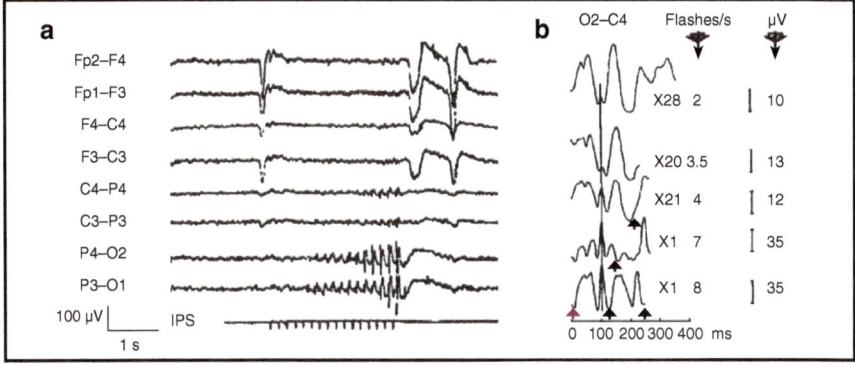

Occipital spikes and their relation to the P_{100} component of the visual-evoked response (VER) in photosensitive patients with generalised PPR

Fig. 1.4 (**a**) Patterned IPS (2×2 mm graticule superimposed on the glass of the stroboscope) evoked occipital spikes, which are time-locked to flash at 6 flashes/s of a patient with spontaneous and photically elicited GTCSs. Higher flash frequencies of 9–30 Hz elicited generalised PPRs of spike–wave, briefly preceded by occipital spikes.[64] (**b**) Emergence of occipital spikes from the P_{100} VER component with increasing flash rate. The patient had spontaneous and television-induced GTCS. On the EEG, time-locked occipital spikes were apparent only at 5 flashes/s, while higher flash rates of 6–26 Hz elicited generalised discharges of spike–wave briefly preceded by occipital spikes. The three upper traces show the average VERs to 2, 3.5 and 4 flashes/s. The occipital spikes evoked at 7 and 8 flashes/s (black arrows) are shown in the two lower traces. The vertical line crosses the negative component of the occipital spikes and the Vb component of the P_{100} component of the VER. The horizontal line indicates time in ms. The *red arrow* indicates the onset of flash (Modified with permission from Panayiotopoulos et al.[70])

- *Posterior (temporoparieto-occipital with occipital emphasis) spike/ polyspike–waves:* This is the mildest form of PPRs and does not spread to the anterior regions. It consists of occipital spikes, polyspikes or slow waves mixed with small, larval spikes (Figs. 1.3 and 1.4). Occipital spikes are often time-locked to the flash with a latency of approximately 100 ms, coinciding with the positive P_{100} of the visual evoked response (Fig. 1.4).[63] Half the patients with posterior PPRs have epileptic seizures (spontaneous, photically elicited or both).[13]

Ictal clinical manifestations during PPRs may be one of the most important factors with regard to risk of seizures, but this has not been studied and emphasised in expert consensus.[95,96]

Fig. 1.3 (**a**) Generalised 3–4 Hz spike/polyspike–waves associated with an absence. The discharge outlasts the duration of the stimulus. (**b**) Generalised polyspike discharge in a patient with symptomatic spontaneous and photically induced seizures, mainly GTCSs, which are resistant to appropriate anti-epileptic medication. This type of discharge is usually associated with myoclonic jerks, which did not feature in this case. Note that the discharge occurs only after eye blinks or eye closure, and does not outlast the stimulus train. (**c**) Typical occipital spikes time-locked to each flash of IPS. The patient is a woman with idiopathic occipital epilepsy (probably a variant of idiopathic childhood occipital epilepsy of Gastaut), who never had attacks precipitated by lights (case report in Agathonikou et al.[99])

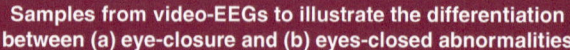

Samples from video-EEGs to illustrate the differentiation between (a) eye-closure and (b) eyes-closed abnormalities

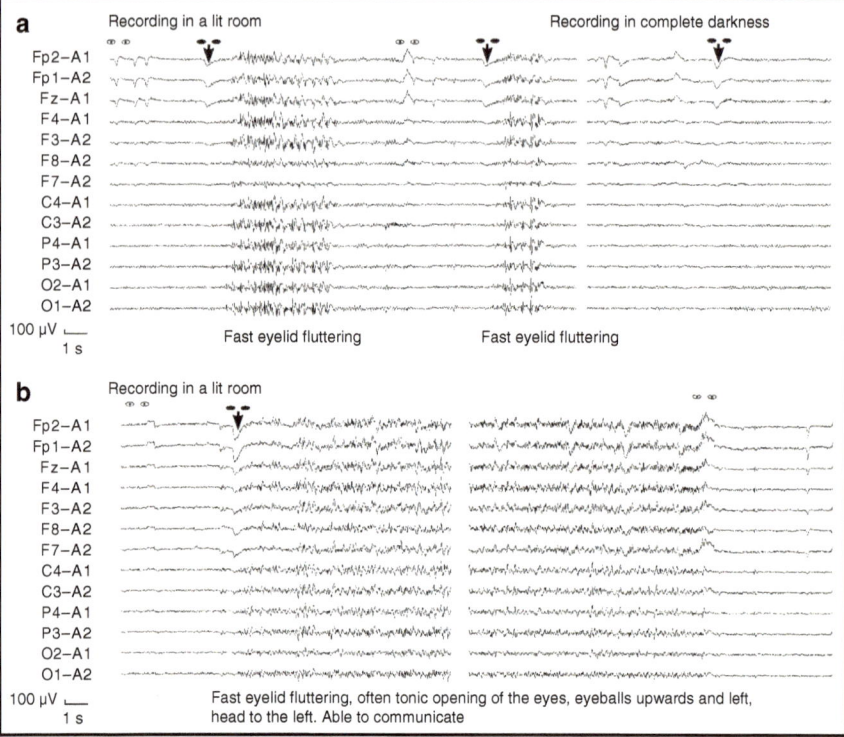

Fig. 1.5 (**a**) Eye-closure-related abnormalities in a patient with Jeavons syndrome.[101] High-amplitude, generalised discharges occur within 1–3 s of closing the eyes in a lit room. These are of brief duration, do not continue in the resting period that the eyes are closed and are totally inhibited in complete darkness. (**b**) Eyes closed-related abnormalities in a woman who probably has cryptogenic epilepsy with seizures related to FOS.[36,102] The EEG paroxysms last as long as the eyes are closed. They are abruptly inhibited when the eyes are opened. The response to fixation-off and fixation-on were similar, irrespective of the means by which they were elicited (eyes closed, darkness, +10 spherical lenses, Ganzfeld stimulation). The best practical means for testing FOS is with underwater goggles covered with opaque tape

Clarification

The effectiveness of eyes open, eyes closed and eye closure during IPS

The state of the eyes during IPS is probably the most significant internal factor that modifies the response to IPS (Figs. 1.3 and 1.5).[100] Eye closure (closing of the eyes while IPS continues) is by far the most potent.[13,100] Of the other two states, eyes open is more susceptible than eyes closed to patterned flickering lights. Conversely, eyes closed appears to be more susceptible than eyes open to direct unpatterned light, probably because of a diffusion effect of light by the eyelids. When light with a diffuser is applied, eyes open is again more effective than eyes closed because of an intensity loss by the closed eyelids.

Clinical Note

Differentiation between eye-closure and eyes-closed state (Fig. 1.5)

Eye closure is the transient state that immediately follows the closing of the eyes, lasts less than 3 s and does not persist in the remaining period of eyes closed. Eye closure is much more potent than 'eyes open' or 'eyes closed' in inducing abnormalities during IPS. Jeavons syndrome is a typical example of eye closure-related seizures and EEG abnormalities. In some photosensitive patients, PPRs occur only after eye closure.

Eyes closed is the state that lasts as long as the eyes remain closed. FOS is a typical example of eyes closed-related seizures and EEG abnormalities.

The resting EEG of patients with idiopathic photic reflex seizures is usually normal or frequently (20–30%) shows eye closure-related paroxysms occurring within 1–3 s after closing of the eyes. These are usually brief EEG paroxysms lasting for 1–4 s and have similar features to those elicited by IPS for each individual patient. They disappear if eye closure occurs in total darkness.

Prognosis

Prognosis is usually good but varies significantly in accordance with the type of photosensitivity. It may be excellent with only one clinical epileptic seizure or be severe with continuing lifelong seizures.[89] Photosensitivity generally declines after the age of 30–40 years.[103]

Management[13]

Avoidance or Prevention of the Provocative Stimulus May Be the Only Treatment

In pure photosensitive seizures, avoidance of the provocative stimulus may be adequate, e.g. patients with television-induced seizures should be advised to view television in a well-lit room, maintain a maximum comfortable viewing distance (typically >2.5 m for a 19-in. screen), use the remote control and – if it is necessary to approach the screen – cover one eye with the palm and avoid prolonged watching, particularly if sleep deprived or tired. Occlusion of one eye is also advised when photosensitive individuals are suddenly exposed to flickering lights such as in discotheques.

Patients with video game-induced seizures should attempt to go without video games, or the time of playing should be significantly restricted and confined to periods when patients are not sleep deprived.

Conditioning treatment or wearing appropriately tinted glasses[104] has been recommended. A new commercially available blue lens, named Z1, was found to be highly effective in controlling PPRs in photosensitive epilepsy patients.[105]

AED Treatment

AED prophylactic treatment is needed for patients with continuing photically induced seizures and for those who also have spontaneous epileptic seizures. The choice of an AED depends on their specific efficacy on photosensitivity, the type/types of reflex and spontaneous seizures, and the particular epileptic syndrome 83a.

Valproate, levetiracetam, lamotrigine and clonazepam suppress photosensitivity in that order of efficacy.[106]

Valproate is effective for all types of photically or spontaneously induced seizure.

Levetiracetam is effective for all types of photically or spontaneously induced seizures. It is very much more efficacious in myoclonic and GTCS than absence seizures.

Lamotrigine is effective for all but myoclonic types of photically or spontaneously induced seizure. Its efficacy in PPRs has been studied mainly with valproate[107] and may be due to their pharmacodynamic interaction. Lamotrigine may be particularly useful in absence seizures when valproate is ineffective or undesirable.

Clonazepam is effective in photically or spontaneously induced myoclonic seizures (but is ineffective against and may exaggerate GTCSs).

Brivaracetam (UCB-34714) is a new AED that has been granted orphan medicinal designation in Europe for the treatment of progressive myoclonic epilepsies and by the FDA in the treatment of symptomatic myoclonus. It has high efficacy in PPRs, which are reduced or abolished in all tested doses (10–80 mg).[108]

Most of the other AEDs (i.e. carbamazepine, gabapentin, oxcarbazepine, phenytoin, pregabalin, tiagabine and vigabatrin) are contraindicated either because:

- They are ineffective (i.e. they induce side effects without providing any therapeutic benefit in addition to depriving patients of appropriate AED treatment)
- They may worsen the seizures.

Idiopathic Photosensitive Occipital Lobe Epilepsy

Idiopathic photosensitive occipital lobe epilepsy (IPOE)[5,12,73,75,109,110] manifests with focal seizures of occipital lobe origin, which are elicited by photic stimuli.

Clarifications on Classification

Occipital seizures precipitated by photic stimuli were overshadowed in the 1989 ILAE classification by the prevailing view that photosensitive epilepsies are mainly generalised.[4] The new ILAE diagnostic scheme[5] recognised IPOE as a new syndrome of reflex epilepsy with age-related onset. This is also maintained in the new ILAE report but with less certainty; IPOE was rated 2 on a score of 1–3 (3 being the most clearly and reproducibly defined) indicating the certainty with which the ILAE Core Group believed that each syndrome represented a unique diagnostic entity.[6]

The boundaries of this syndrome of IPOE are genuinely uncertain. OPSs may start in adulthood, be part of idiopathic childhood occipital epilepsy of Gastaut (ICOE-G),[111] develop later in children with rolandic seizures or occur accidentally during IPS of normal individuals or those with migraine.[12,109] Gastaut[111] included IPOE in his syndrome:

- Seven of 63 patients had IPS evoked occipital spikes, 'not seen in the resting EEG' and 'unrelated to eye opening and closing'.
- Seven other patients with typical occipital paroxysms had generalised PPRs, which sometimes were associated with myoclonus (see also case 11 in Gaustaut et al.[111]).

Contrary to this is the view that 'reflex triggering of seizures have not been reported' in ICOE-G.[75]

Depending on severity, there may be three significant groups of OPSs:[12,109]

1. OPSs may occur in patients with a low occipital epileptogenic threshold to IPS that manifests with seizures only under extreme exposure to the offending stimulation. These are 'seizures that do not require a diagnosis of epilepsy'.[5] Accidental single isolated occipital seizures in normal young people[112] or patients with migraine[112] during IPS are most likely, due to a low threshold to such events, and may not happen again.
2. OPSs in patients with idiopathic occipital epileptogenicity, which probably constitute the major part of IPOE. Patients, usually children, have clinical PPRs elicited by various environmental light stimulation (video games are far more common than television).

C.P. Panayiotopoulos, *Reflex Seizures and Related Epileptic Syndromes*, DOI 10.1007/978-1-4471-4042-9_2, © Springer-Verlag London 2012

3. OPSs occurring in patients, usually children, with idiopathic focal or generalised epilepsies other than IPOE. These are often demanding cases with regard to diagnosis and management.

4. OPSs with bizarre ictal symptomatology mimicking hysterical attacks or migraine are well reported.[12] That these symptoms, even the very prolonged and unusual ones, are ictal has been documented with ictal EEGs.[73]

Considering all of these, the data presented in this chapter may not accurately represent a single syndrome of IPOE.

Demographic Data[109,113]

Onset of the first provoked seizure may range from 15 months to adulthood (peak 12–14 years). Whether females predominate[110,113] is debatable.[109] Prevalence is reported as low, at around 0.4% of all epilepsies.[109] However, OPSs reached epidemic proportions in Japan among children watching the animated cartoon television programme *Pokémon* (*Pocket Monsters*).[74]

Clinical Manifestations[12,73,75,109,110]

Occipital seizures precipitated by photic stimuli are induced by video games and less often by television or other photic stimuli. These reflex seizures contain all the elements detailed in the spontaneous seizures of occipital lobe epilepsy.[73,114-116] OPSs commonly manifest with visual hallucinations, blurring of vision or blindness, alone or in combination. Less often, these visual symptoms may follow other ictal occipital manifestations, such as deviation of the eyes and head, eyelid fluttering and orbital pain.

Visual symptoms may be the only ictal manifestations, usually lasting for seconds and frequently 1–3 min. When longer (5–15 min), other ictal manifestations also occur.[73,114] Consciousness is not impaired during the phase of visual symptoms.

Progression of visual seizures to other ictal symptoms: Autonomic symptoms, such as those occurring in Panayiotopoulos syndrome (mainly retching and ictal vomiting), often follow the occipital symptoms and may end with secondarily GTCSs.[73,75]

Other type of seizures: Patients with IPOE may have exclusively OPSs. Others may also have spontaneous visual or other types of seizures. These vary from eyelid fluttering, myoclonic jerks and absences to GTCSs that occur independently of the occipital seizures.[109,113] In some cases, spontaneous secondarily GTCSs occur only during sleep.[12] Rarely, patients with rolandic seizures may later develop OPSs.[12,115]

Post-ictal symptoms: OPSs, like the spontaneous occipital seizures, are more likely than any other type of focal seizures to be followed by headache, nausea and vomiting. The headache is usually mild and diffuse, but may also be severe and throbbing, occurring 10–20 min after the end of the visual hallucinations. Post-ictal headache may also be associated with vomiting, lasting for several hours.[73]

Precipitating Factors

By definition, all patients with IPOE are sensitive to flickering lights. Depending on the severity of photosensitivity in some patients, seizures may be elicited by minimal photic provocation; in others, combined pattern and photic or prolonged exposure may be responsible, whereas in others still (probably most cases of IPOE) photic stimuli are effective only if combined with other precipitating factors such as excitement or frustration, fatigue and sleep deprivation.[11]

Diagnostic Procedures

All except the EEG are normal.

Electroencephalography[12,73,75,109,110]

By definition, all these patients are photosensitive and IPS elicits abnormal EEG paroxysms of spikes or polyspikes, which may be entirely confined to

the occipital regions, or PPRs of generalised spike–wave discharges (GSWD), which predominate in the posterior regions (Figs. 2.1 and 2.2). Spontaneous, mainly posterior, spikes often appear in the resting EEG. Centrotemporal spikes may coexist.

Occipital spikes and other posterior abnormalities induced by IPS are considered to be of much lower epileptogenic capacity than generalised PPRs. They may occur in 50% of patients who do not have seizures.[13] Occipital spikes precede generalised PPRs in 90% of photosensitive patients when light and pattern are combined during IPS.[13,117,118]

Ictal EEGs have documented the occipital origin and spreading of the discharges to the temporal regions.[75]

In my experience with video-EEG recordings, most patients with IPOE also have other types of seizure induced by IPS such as eyelid, limb, body or finger myoclonic jerks, eyelid flickering or brief absences that are sometimes mild and may escape detection without video-EEG and if cognition is not tested (Fig. 2.1).[12]

Visual evoked potentials are always of abnormally high amplitude,[75] as indeed they are in any type of photosensitive epilepsy (Fig. 1.3).

Aetiology

By definition, idiopathic photosensitive occipital lobe epilepsy is idiopathic with genetic influences. Some patients have a family history of IPOE or IGE. Overlapping with JME has been reported.[113] Symptomatic occipital photosensitivity[119] is not part of IPOE.

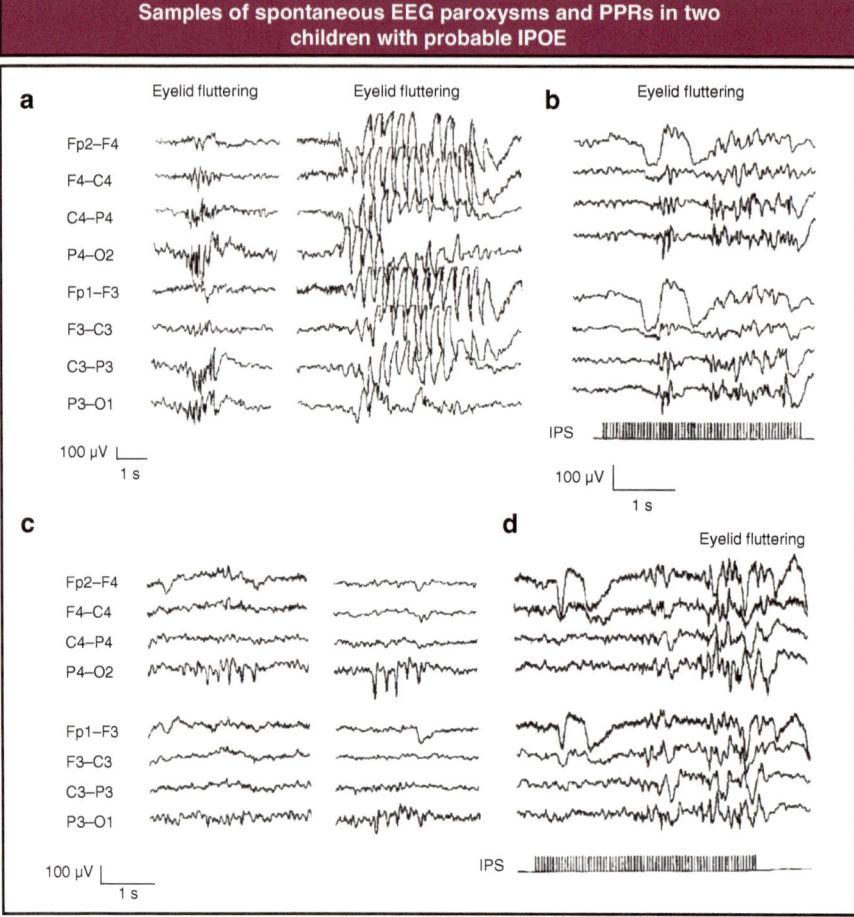

Fig. 2.1 (**a**) Spontaneous occipital spikes/polyspikes and generalised discharges are associated with eyelid fluttering, which is conspicuous on video-EEG. Neither the patient nor her relatives were aware of these. (**b**) IPS consistently elicited posterior spikes, which were also associated with ictal eyelid fluttering. This patient (**a, b**) had typical multicoloured visual seizures from the age of 5 years (case 12.1 in Panayiotopoulos[12]). They were elicited by environmental lights and occasionally progressed to GTCS. She improved over the years but at 20 years of age, while on medication with valproate, she had a visual seizure with GTCS while watching television from a nearly touching distance. High-resolution MRI was normal. (**c**) Spontaneous occipital paroxysms without discernible clinical manifestations. (**d**) IPS consistently elicited PPRs with maximum posterior emphasis. These were often associated with conspicuous eyelid fluttering. This patient (**c, d**) illustrates the links between IPOE and the benign childhood seizure susceptibility syndrome (case 12.2 in Panayiotopoulos[12]). She initially had typical rolandic seizures and then developed frequent visual seizures, often with secondarily GTCSs. These were sometimes photically induced, but more often occurred during sleep. High-resolution MRI was normal

Differential Diagnosis

The differential diagnosis of IPOE includes migraine (rarely an actual problem if symptoms are appropriately analysed), ICOE-G, IGE (probably of management importance) and non-epileptic paroxysmal events (sometimes very difficult to differentiate).

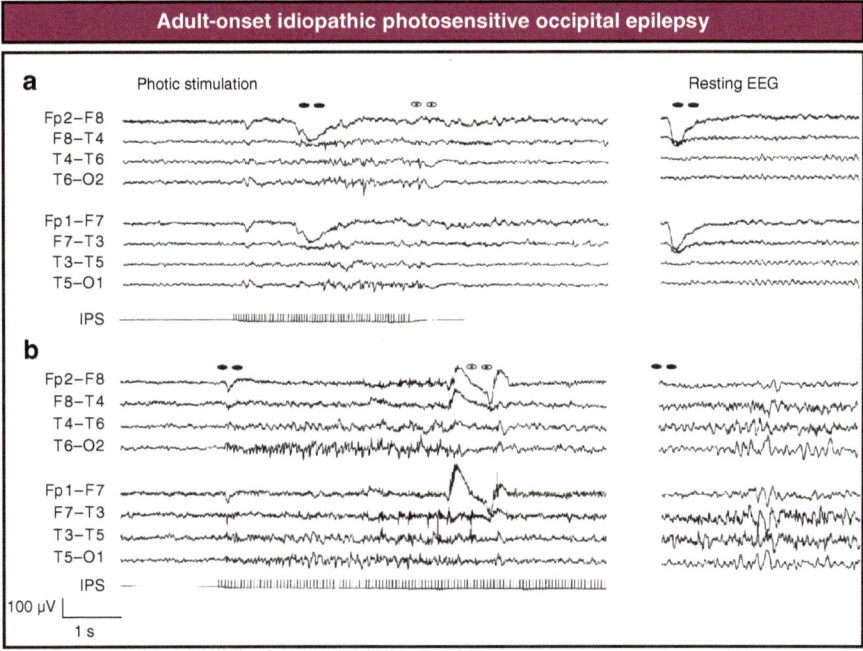

Fig. 2.2 (**a**) Sample from an EEG of a man who had his first seizure at the age of 35 years while in a lift cradle at work. His vision became blurred, he felt dizzy and, within 2 min, he had a GTCS. No further seizures occurred in the next 6 months of follow-up. MRI was normal. (**b**) Sample from an EEG of a woman who had her first seizure at the age of 31 years. There was a cluster of precipitating factors; she had consumed a few alcoholic drinks, was sleep deprived, 4 months pregnant and dancing exposed to flickering discotheque lights until the early hours of the next day. She first experienced whirling lights in front of her eyes, visual perception became disturbed and within 1 min she had a GTCS. She was well during the next 4 months of follow-up. MRI was normal

The differential diagnosis of visual seizures from all types of migraine with visual aura has been detailed elsewhere. Some seizures of IPOE may be prolonged, also progressing from visual symptoms to nausea and vomiting with altered consciousness.[73,120] The spread of the discharge from the occipital cortex can be slow, and responsiveness may be maintained while the patient is vomiting.[73,120] These seizures may be erroneously diagnosed as migraine proper.

In children and adolescents, the differentiation of IPOE from ICOE-G may not be needed if they are the same syndrome.

Differentiation of IPOE from generalised photosensitive epilepsies should rely on clinical criteria. Occipital spikes often precede generalised discharges in photosensitive epilepsies.

In adults we have reported occipital photosensitivity in adult patients aged about 30 who presented with a late-onset first GTCS (often preceded by visual symptoms).[121] Of 1,550 patients with seizures, three women and two men (0.3%) had EEG occipital photosensitivity and onset of solitary (three patients) or infrequent seizures in adulthood (median age 31 years, range 26–35 years).

All five of these patients had generalised convulsions, which were preceded by blurring of vision or elementary visual hallucinations in four cases. Precipitation by lights, alone or in combination with other factors, was apparent in only two patients. Seizures were diurnal in all but one patient. According to the inclusion criteria, all patients had EEG occipital spikes elicited by IPS (Fig. 2.2). Neurological and intellectual states, as well as brain imaging, were normal.

Prognosis[12,73,75,109,110]

Frequency of seizures and overall prognosis vary significantly among affected individuals. This depends on the severity of photosensitivity and exposure to the offending visual stimuli. There are rare case reports of normal young people[112] or patients with migraine[112,122] having an occipital seizure during IPS.

Some patients may have only one or two occipital seizures in their life despite exposure to precipitating factors and no drug treatment.[12,73,75] Others, particularly those who also have spontaneous seizures, may need medication for 1–3 years, together with strict avoidance of or cautious exposure to insulting stimuli. However, other patients may have frequent spontaneous and elicited occipital fits alone or in combination with other types of seizures, which include myoclonic jerks, often of the eyelids, infrequent absences or GTCSs.[12]

Management

Advice about avoidance of precipitating factors is essential and is similar to that given to patients with any type of photosensitivity. Particular emphasis is needed about video games and television. Commercially available blue lenses, named Z1, that are highly effective in controlling PPRs[105] may be of value.

The effectiveness of valproate has not been tested in OPSs as it has in generalised photosensitive seizures. Patients with IPOE who are resistant to valproate became seizure free with add-on carbamazepine.[12,99] Levetiracetam or clobazam are possible alternatives 83a.

Jeavons Syndrome

Synonym: eyelid myoclonia with absences.

Jeavons syndrome[101,109,123-129] is one of the most distinctive reflex IGE syndromes characterised by the triad of:

- Eyelid myoclonia with and without absences
- Eye closure-induced seizures, EEG paroxysms or both
- Photosensitivity

Considerations on Classification

Jeavons syndrome refers to an *idiopathic reflex epilepsy*, which has unique clinical and EEG features; eyelid myoclonia is the defining seizure type. The ILAE has not yet recognised Jeavons syndrome despite overwhelming evidence.[101,109,123-129] Instead, 'eyelid myoclonia' has been accepted as a unique seizure entity with the comment that 'the degree to which these recurrent events (5 or 6 Hz) are associated with impairment of consciousness has not been adequately documented, and should be. In some patients they can be provoked by eye closure'.[6] However, it is well established that eyelid myoclonia may occur:

- With and without absences (see the clinical manifestations below)
- In many epileptic conditions of idiopathic (Jeavons syndrome), symptomatic or probably symptomatic causes[129]

Whether or not their pathophysiology and anatomical substrates are distinct (to constitute a unique seizure diagnostic entity)[6] is unknown.

Demographic Data[101,109]

Onset is typically in childhood with a peak at age 6–8 years (range 2–14 years). There is a twofold preponderance of girls. The prevalence of Jeavons syndrome is around 3% among adult patients with epileptic disorders and 13% among those with IGEs with absences.[101]

Clinical Manifestations

Eyelid myoclonia, not the absences, is the hallmark of Jeavons syndrome (Figs. 1.4 and 3.1).

Eyelid myoclonia consists of marked jerking of the eyelids often associated with jerky upwards deviation of the eyeballs and retropulsion of the head

C.P. Panayiotopoulos, *Reflex Seizures and Related Epileptic Syndromes*, 21
DOI 10.1007/978-1-4471-4042-9_3, © Springer-Verlag London 2012

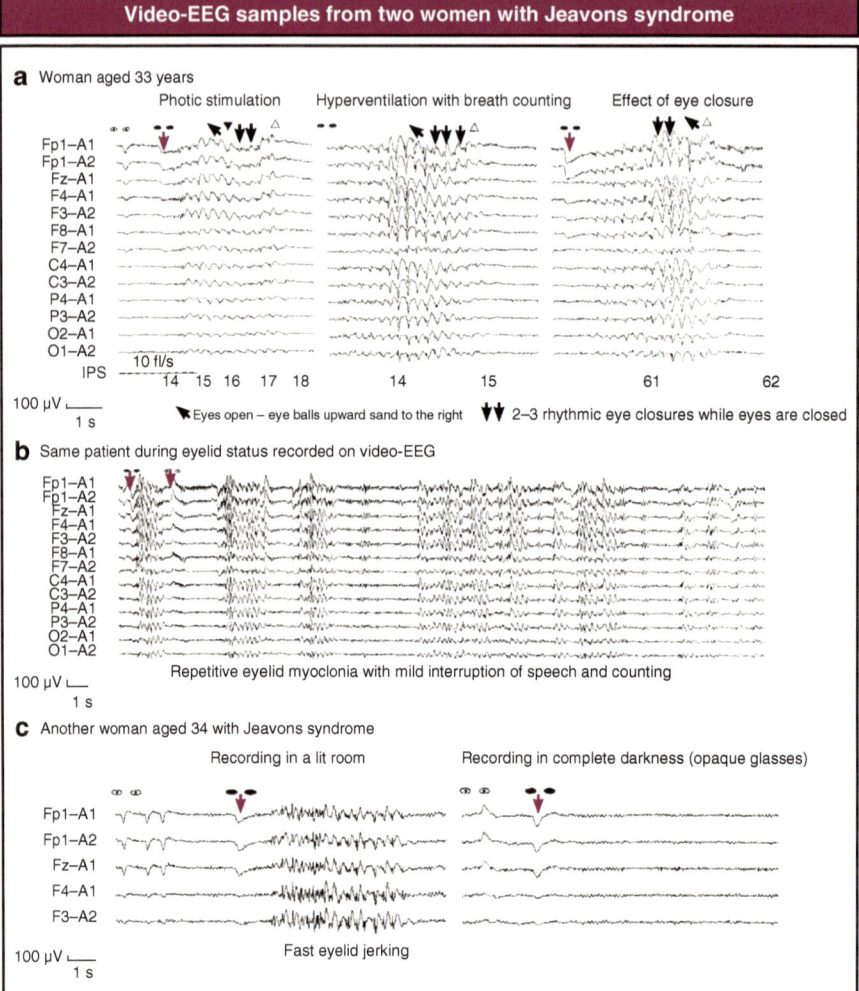

Fig. 3.1 (**a**) Brief GSWD with similar characteristics are induced by IPS (*left*) or eye closure (*right*). They occasionally occur spontaneously (*middle*). In all illustrated occasions, these GSWD were associated with marked eyelid myoclonia denoted by the *black arrows*. Also note that there is no impairment of counting (numbers). (**b**) Repetitive discontinuous seizures of eyelid myoclonia occurred on awakening when the patient was erroneously treated with carbamazepine. These lasted for more than 30 min. There was only mild interruption of speech and counting during the GSWD. The patient was fully aware of her condition. (**c**) Long video-EEG of a woman with Jeavons syndrome while taking valproate. There were frequent eye-closure-related GSWD of mainly polyspikes, often associated with fast eyelid jerking, which could be mild or violent. They were totally inhibited in complete darkness (complete darkness implies that any form of possible light was totally eliminated). Symbols of eyes indicate when the eyes were open or closed. Video-EEG samples of these and other patients with Jeavons syndrome can be seen in the CD companion of references[57-59]

(eyelid myoclonia *without* absences). This may be associated with or followed by mild impairment of consciousness (eyelid myoclonia *with* absences). The seizures are brief (3–6 s) and occur mainly after eye closure and consistently many times a day. All patients are photosensitive.

GTCSs, either induced by lights or spontaneous, are probably inevitable in the long term and are provoked particularly by precipitating factors (sleep deprivation, alcohol) and inappropriate AED modifications. Typically, GTCSs are sparse and avoidable.

Myoclonic jerks of the limbs may occur, but are infrequent and random.

Eyelid myoclonic status epilepticus, either spontaneous (mainly on awakening) or photically induced, occurs in a fifth of patients. It consists of repetitive and discontinuous episodes of eyelid myoclonia with mild absence, rather than continuous non-convulsive absence status epilepticus (Fig. 3.1).

Precipitating Factors

The most potent precipitating factor is eye closure, whether voluntary, involuntary or reflex. Most and, in some patients, all of the seizures are induced immediately after closure of the eyes in the presence of uninterrupted (non-flickering) light. Eye closure in total darkness is ineffective.

Contrary to other forms of photosensitive epilepsies that are sensitive only to flickering lights (IPS), patients with Jeavons syndrome are also sensitive to bright, non-flickering lights. This is probably due to the enhancing effect of bright light on the sensitivity of eye closure.

Self-induction in Jeavons Syndrome

Most relevant reports and the majority of epileptologists unquestionably consider the eyelid myoclonia of Jeavons syndrome as a manoeuvre used by patients to self-induce IPS and elicit seizures (see Misconceptions). My view, based on numerous video-EEG recordings and interviews with 17 patients, is that eyelid myoclonia is an ictal event (15 patients) and that self-induced seizures in Jeavons syndrome are rare (possibly two patients).[85] After all, these patients do not need IPS to induce seizures. Closing the eyes (there is no need for forceful slow eye closure) in the presence of uninterrupted light may be more powerful than IPS in provoking a seizure. In physiological terms, these clinical manifestations are likely to be similar to an 'attraction movement' to light and other manifestations of the 'optic fixation reflexes', when volitional movements of the eyes are unattainable or weak.[130]

My eyes flicker as a reflex to the light.

Patients consider eyelid myoclonia as a socially embarrassing condition, they are relieved when the seizures improve with AEDs and they show excellent compliance with their treatment.

It has been proposed that patients with Jeavons syndrome may not be deliberate 'self-inducers', but may suffer from compulsive 'self-induction' similar to the phenomenology of Tourette syndrome.[124] This is because some patients may have various compulsive or tic-like symptoms, including premonitory sensations, compulsive and difficult-to-resist urges and a sense of relief associated with the attacks.[124]

Aetiology

Jeavons syndrome is a genetically determined homogeneous syndrome, with a high prevalence of similar seizures in family members.[131,132]

Pathophysiology

It is possible that in patients with Jeavons syndrome the α-rhythm generators malfunction, and that both the magnocellular and parvocellular systems are functionally disturbed. We do not know the physiology of the epileptic phenomena and the alterations that may occur in the brain of patients with Jeavons syndrome, under the continuous bombardment from electrical discharges almost every time that they close their eyes. Age at onset may be significant.

Diagnostic Procedures

All tests apart from the EEG are normal.

Electroencephalography

Video-EEG is the single most important procedure for the diagnosis of eyelid myoclonia with or without absences. It shows frequent high-amplitude 3–6 Hz GSWD of mainly polyspikes (Figs. 1.4 and 3.1). Typically these are:

- Related to eye closure, i.e. they occur immediately (within 0.5–2 s) on closing the eyes in an illuminated recording room and they are eliminated in total darkness
- Brief (1–6 s, commonly 2 or 3 s)

GSWD are also enhanced by hyperventilation. Eyelid myoclonia of varying severity often occurs with GSWD.

PPRs are recorded in all untreated young patients, but may be absent in older patients or those on medication. Photosensitivity and FOS may coexist.

Sleep EEG patterns are normal. GSWD are more likely to increase during sleep, but may also decrease. In sleep, the GSWD are shorter and devoid of discernible clinical manifestations of any type, even in those patients who have numerous seizures during alert states.

The EEG and clinical manifestations deteriorate consistently after awakening.

A normal EEG is rare, even in well-controlled patients.

Differential Diagnosis

The diagnosis of Jeavons syndrome is simple because the characteristic eyelid myoclonia, if seen once, will never be forgotten or confused with other conditions.[109] Furthermore, the EEG with the characteristic eye-closure-related discharges and photosensitivity leaves no room for diagnostic error.

As a simple rule of thumb, eyelid myoclonia is highly suggestive of Jeavons syndrome. This becomes more likely when eyelid myoclonia is combined with photosensitivity, and it is pathognomonic of the syndrome when it also occurs after eye closure.

Nevertheless, eyelid myoclonia is often misdiagnosed as facial tics, sometimes for many years. In addition, eyelid myoclonia should not be confused with either of the following:

- The rhythmic or random closing of the eyes, often seen in other forms of IGE with absences
- The eyelid jerking that may occur at the opening or initial stage of the GSWD in typical absence seizures of childhood absence epilepsy

Persistent, frequent, non-epileptic, paroxysmal eyelid movements that occur in patients with PPRs are a source of diagnostic confusion that can be avoided with video-EEG recordings.[133]

The main diagnostic problem, which is probably iatrogenic, is self-induction. This is a diagnosis that should not be made without taking a proper history because it is often wrong (see misconceptions below).

The symptom/seizure of eyelid myoclonia alone is not sufficient to characterise Jeavons syndrome, as it may also occur in symptomatic and cryptogenic epilepsies, which are betrayed by developmental delay, learning difficulties, neurological deficits, and abnormal MRI and background EEG.[134]

Misconceptions

A main misconception is that eyelid myoclonia (the seizure) is a self-induced attempt to induce seizures. This belief is so strong that, in almost all relevant publications, the patient described by Radovici et al.[135] is erroneously cited as the first reported case of self-induced seizures, even by hand waving.[86] No such evidence or mention of self-induced seizures can be found in the original report: 'AA… age de 20 ans, presente des troubles moteurs sous forme de mouvements involontaires de la tête et des yeux sous l'influence des rayons solaires.'[135]

Prognosis

Jeavons syndrome is a lifelong disorder, even if seizures are well controlled with AEDs. Men have a better prognosis than women. There is a tendency for photosensitivity to disappear in middle age, but eyelid myoclonia persists. It is highly resistant to treatment and occurs many times a day, often without apparent absences and even without demonstrable photosensitivity.

Management[109,129]

Based on anecdotal evidence, the drugs of choice are those used for other IGEs 83a.

Valproate alone, or most probably in combination with clonazepam, levetiracetam, lamotrigine or ethosuximide, appears to be the most effective regimen. The choice of the second drug depends on the main seizure type. Clonazepam is highly efficacious in eyelid myoclonia and myoclonic jerks; some patients achieve relatively good control with clonazepam monotherapy.

Of the newer AEDs, levetiracetam may be the most effective, because of its antimyoclonic and antiphotosensitive properties. Lamotrigine is very effective in absence seizures but may exaggerate myoclonic jerks.

Carbamazepine, gabapentin, oxcarbazepine, phenytoin, pregabalin, tiagabine and vigabatrin are contraindicated.

Lifestyle and avoidance of seizure precipitants are important.

Non-pharmacological treatments used for photosensitive patients (such as wearing special glasses or the newly commercially available blue Z1 lenses) should be employed in Jeavons syndrome when photosensitivity persists.[105,136]

Pattern-Sensitive Epilepsy

Pattern-sensitive epilepsy[13,14,33,34,77,137,138] refers to epileptic seizures induced by patterns; it is not a particular epileptic syndrome. Pattern seizure sensitivity is closely related to photosensitivity. Almost all patients with clinical pattern sensitivity epilepsy show PPRs (Figs. 4.1 and 4.2). Conversely, 30% of clinically photosensitive patients are also sensitive to stationary, and 70% to appropriately vibrating, patterns of stripes. Patterns enhance the effect of photic stimulation, whether under test conditions or in real life. Pattern sensitivity without photosensitivity, sensitivity to non-geometric patterns and self-induced pattern-sensitive epilepsy are all rare.

Demographic Data

Pure pattern-sensitive epilepsy with clinical attacks induced only by patterns is rare[34]; it probably occurs in 0.2% of patients with onset of non-febrile seizures between birth and 15 years of age.[109] This is despite the relatively high incidence of pattern-induced EEG paroxysmal activity in photosensitive patients.

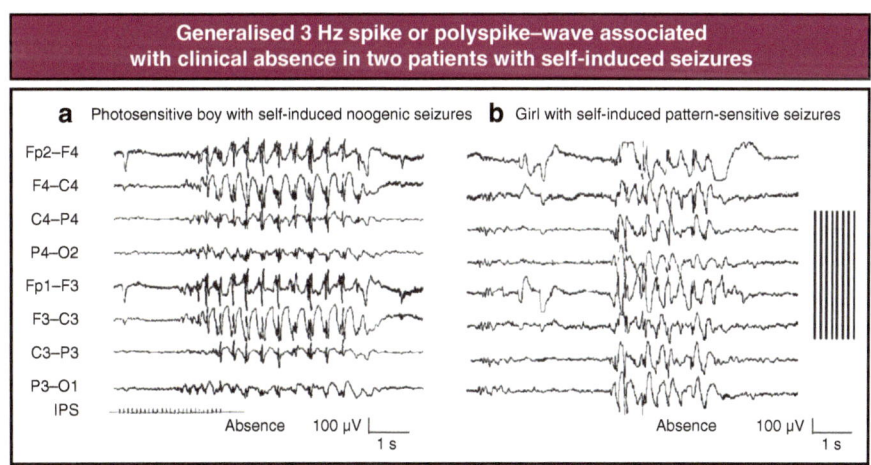

Generalised 3 Hz spike or polyspike–wave associated with clinical absence in two patients with self-induced seizures

a Photosensitive boy with self-induced noogenic seizures **b** Girl with self-induced pattern-sensitive seizures

Fp2–F4, F4–C4, C4–P4, P4–O2, Fp1–F3, F3–C3, C3–P3, P3–O1, IPS

Absence 100 μV 1 s

Absence 100 μV 1 s

Fig. 4.1 (**a**) Absence seizure induced by IPS. This patient had spontaneous, photically induced and noogenic seizures. He used noogenic processes for self-induction (see Koutroumanidis et al.[51]). (**b**) Absence seizure induced by a pattern with vertical lines. This patient with learning difficulties had mainly self-induced pattern-sensitive epilepsy. She was also photosensitive (see Panayiotopoulos[35]) (Modified with permission from Koutroumanidis et al.[51] and Panayiotopoulos[35])

C.P. Panayiotopoulos, *Reflex Seizures and Related Epileptic Syndromes*,
DOI 10.1007/978-1-4471-4042-9_4, © Springer-Verlag London 2012

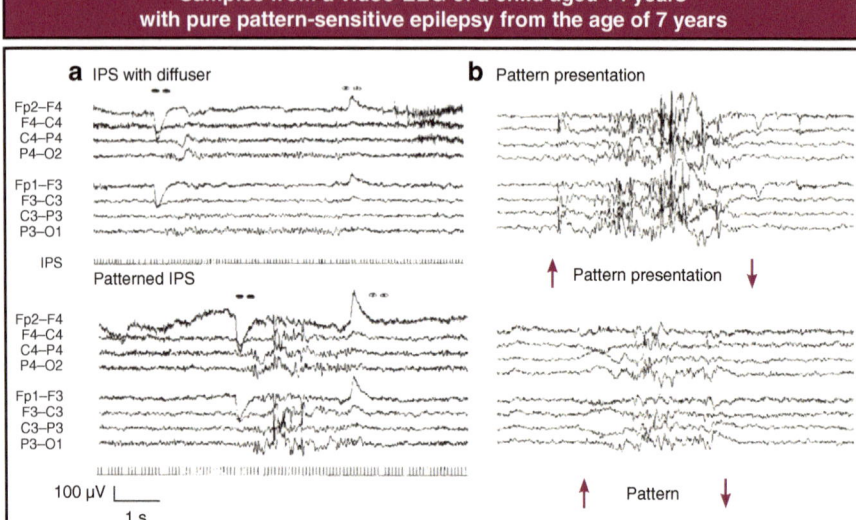

Fig. 4.2 (**a**) Only patterned IPS (2×2 mm graticule superimposed on the glass of the stroboscope)[64,97] elicits PPRs. (**b**) Paroxysmal discharges were consistently elicited by various linear patterns. The child is of normal development and scholastic performance. He has brief 4–10 s absence seizures consisting of mild-to-moderate impairment of consciousness and concurrent upwards rolling of the eyeballs with eyelid flickering. The seizures are invariably elicited by patterns with grids or stripes, such as escalators, and the dotted lines of microwaves, radiators or cloths. On five occasions, the absence seizures were followed by GTCSs. He is also drawn like a magnet to the television screen, although he is not photosensitive. Spontaneous absence seizures occur only after awakening. A characteristic feature is that when patterns appear in his visual field, his eyes fixate (freeze) to them and he is unable to turn away. He says that he finds patterns 'hypnotic', but not pleasant. He would avoid patterns if he could and does not seek them out. This behaviour was considered as 'self-induction', but this was not the opinion shared by Dr. A. Wilkins (a renowned expert in pattern and photosensitive epilepsies) and myself who examined him together

Clinical Manifestations

Clinical manifestations have not been well studied in pure pattern-sensitive epilepsy.[13,34] All types of generalised seizures have been described. My impression is that absences are more common than GTCSs and myoclonic jerks, and GTCSs are more common than myoclonic jerks. I am not aware of patterns inducing occipital seizures, although they should exist considering that the visual cortex is the primary target of the pattern stimulus. Self-induced pattern-sensitive epilepsy has been reported (Fig. 4.1).[35,139]

Environmental Stimuli

Environmental stimuli that induce seizures in pattern-sensitive patients are those that best match the properties of the provocative patterns used in relevant EEG testing, and best suit and create the conditions of their spatial and directional presentation to the eyes. These are striped clothes, such as shirts, jackets or ties, and escalators, wallpaper and furnishings, Venetian blinds, air-conditioning grills and radiators. Any activity visually involved with these patterns, such as ironing, is likely to induce seizures. Less direct, but often very significant, is the role of patterns in more complex stimuli, such as television viewing and video games.[13,14,33]

Patients, caregivers and physicians recognise pattern as a seizure precipitant less often than environmental flicker or specific agents, such as the television, discotheque lighting or video games. Direct questioning implicates pattern as a seizure trigger in 6–30%[82,140] of photosensitive individuals.

Aetiology

Pattern sensitivity, similar to photosensitive epilepsy, is a genetically determined trait.

Pathophysiology

Elaborate and intelligent methodological studies, mainly in patients with photically induced seizures, revealed many aspects of pattern seizure susceptibility and its pathophysiology[14,33]:

- Seizures are triggered in the visual cortex
- Synchronisation of neural activity is necessary
- The trigger involves one cerebral hemisphere or both hemispheres independently
- The trigger requires the physiological activation of a critical area of cortical tissue

Diagnostic Procedures

The EEG with appropriate pattern presentations is the key test (Fig. 4.2). Pattern sensitivity depends on the spatial frequency, orientation, brightness, contrast and size of the pattern. An optimally epileptogenic pattern consists of black-and-white stripes of equal width and spacing (see the literature[14,33,109]). As in photosensitive patients, binocular is much more potent than monocular stimulation, and the patient should fixate on the presenting patterns.

Prognosis

The prognosis of pattern-sensitive epilepsy has not been systematically studied but may be worse than that of photosensitive epilepsy.

Management

Management may be similar to that of photosensitive epilepsy, but pattern-sensitive epilepsy may be much more difficult to treat.

Fixation-off Sensitivity

5

FOS is a term that I coined to denote the form(s) of epilepsy and/or EEG abnormalities that are elicited by elimination of central vision and fixation.[36,102,109] 'Elimination of central vision and fixation' is a specific precipitating stimulus, which, even in the presence of light, induces high-amplitude occipital or generalised paroxysmal discharges.

FOS is suggested in the routine EEG by abnormalities, which consistently occur as long as the eyes are closed, but not when the eyes are opened.

Clinical and EEG Correlations in Patients with FOS

FOS, similar to photosensitivity, is a reflex EEG activation with some preference for certain epileptic conditions.

From clinical and video-EEG documentation, there are three types of patients with seizures and EEG abnormalities of FOS[36]:

1. *Patients with occipital paroxysms* such as those seen in EEGs of some patients with Panayiotopoulos syndrome and more frequently in patients with ICOE-G, which are the model examples of FOS. It was in these cases that FOS was first documented as a new type of activating stimulus in reflex epilepsies (Fig. 5.1).

   FOS-induced abnormalities are mainly localised in the occipital regions and are not associated with overt ictal clinical manifestations.

2. *A rare but 'pure' and distinct clinical form of FOS cryptogenic generalised epilepsy* (Fig. 1.5b). Patients are women of borderline normal intelligence with frequent eyelid myoclonia (with or without *atypical* absences), absence status epilepticus and GTCSs. The eyelid myoclonia manifests with fast, small amplitude clonic movements of the eyelids associated with tonic spasm of the eyelids and eyes that occasionally spread to the neck muscles.[102] Absence status epilepticus is preferentially catamenial.[141]

   Another of our patients also has catamenial absence status epilepticus, 'always coming with her menstruation' every month.[141] This lasts for 1–3 days when 'she is vacant, eyes rolling up, feeling slow, drowsy and depressed but also aggressive and not in control of herself'. She had four to five GTCSs in her life, probably after an absence status and indulgence in alcohol.[141]

C.P. Panayiotopoulos, *Reflex Seizures and Related Epileptic Syndromes*,
DOI 10.1007/978-1-4471-4042-9_5, © Springer-Verlag London 2012

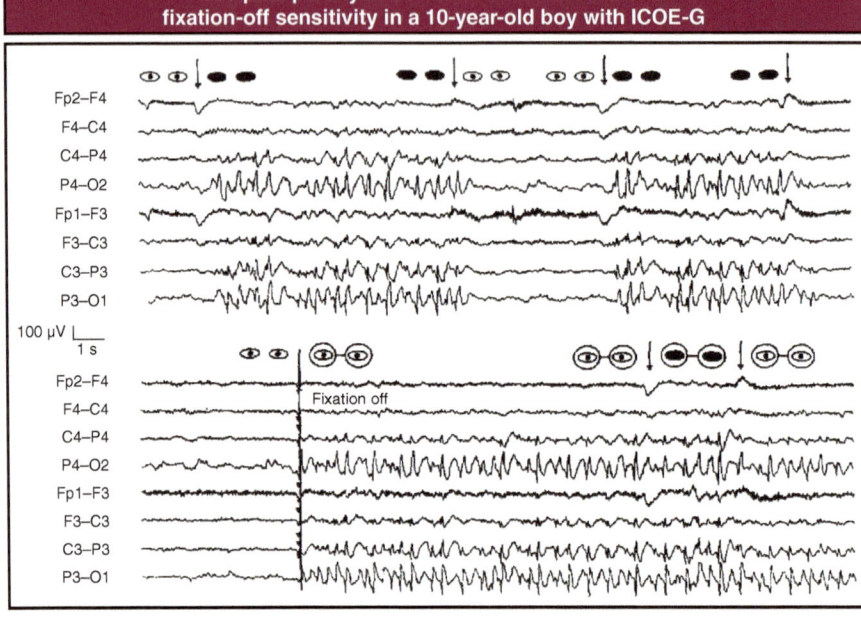

Fig. 5.1 Case 26 in Panayiotopoulos.[1] Occipital paroxysms occur as long as fixation and central vision are eliminated by any means (eyes closed, darkness, +10 spherical lenses, Ganzfeld stimulation). Under these conditions, eye opening cannot inhibit the spikes. Symbols of the eyes open or closed without glasses denote that the recording was made with the lights on and whenever fixation was possible. Symbols of the eyes open or closed with glasses denote that the recording was made when fixation and central vision were eliminated by any of the above means (Reproduced with permission from Panayiotopoulos (1999)[1])

EEG-FOS abnormalities consist mainly of diffuse α-like rhythms at 7 Hz, mixed with bisynchronous sharp and spike/polyspike components. These are often associated with clinical ictal manifestations (Fig. 1.4b). Patients are not photosensitive and differ markedly from those with Jeavons syndrome (eyelid myoclonia with absences).

3. *Patients with IGEs and photosensitivity.*[109,142] The FOS abnormalities are often diffuse and not associated with overt clinical ictal manifestations.

In the second and third types, the typical abnormalities related to FOS are mainly diffuse/generalised, with 'dropout' in sleep stages simultaneous with the α-rhythm.

FOS may occur in individuals without seizures.[143] In an example of such an asymptomatic adult with FOS, continuous bilateral occipital paroxysms during elimination of central vision were associated with transitory cognitive impairment, demonstrated by neuropsychological testing.[143]

The range of EEG abnormalities and clinical manifestations associated with FOS may be extended if FOS is tested as part of routine clinical practice of EEG departments.

	FOS	Photosensitivity
Resting EEG in a lit recording room	Eye-closed abnormalities	Eye-closure abnormalities
Effect of darkness	Activation of abnormalities	Inhibition of abnormalities
Effect of fixation and central vision	Inhibition of abnormalities	Activation of abnormalities
Effect of patterns	Inhibition of abnormalities	Activation of abnormalities
Effect of IPS	None or inhibition	Photoparoxysmal responses

Table 5.1 FOS versus photosensitivity

Pathophysiology

The underlying mechanisms of FOS are not known, but they may be related to an abnormality of the α-rhythm generators.[36]

FOS has the opposite EEG characteristics of photosensitivity epilepsies (Table 5.1), but conversion from one to the other may occur, albeit rarely.[36]

FOS paroxysms studied with functional MRI (fMRI) were correlated with activation of parietooccipital and frontal brain areas,[143] and a significant increase of blood oxygen level-dependent signal in the extrastriate cortex.[144] Magnetoencephalography (MEG) of visual evoked fields in FOS revealed abnormal activation of the visual corticocortical pathway via the insular cortex.[145]

Scotosensitive Epilepsy

Scotosensitivity (*skotos* = darkness) denotes forms of epilepsy, seizures or EEG abnormalities that are elicited by the complete elimination of retinal stimulation by light. Pure scotosensitive patients are rare.[146] Most patients described as scotosensitive probably have FOS.[36]

Techniques for Documenting FOS[36]

First, it is essential to confirm that the EEG abnormalities observed in routine EEG recording are related to the eyes-closed state. The patient is asked to open and close his or her eyes every 5 s, six times consecutively.

Instructing the patient to look at a fixed point, such as the tip of a pencil, ensures fixation in the eyes-opened state.

Important Practical Note

Complete darkness can be difficult to achieve in routine EEG departments. Even a small spot of red light on which the eyes may fixate can totally inhibit EEG abnormalities induced by complete darkness. Switching off the lights in the EEG recording room is not adequate and may explain conflicting results in the literature. Complete darkness can be produced with underwater goggles covered completely with opaque tape.

Second, FOS is evaluated by instructing the patient to perform the same sequence of eyes-opened and eyes-closed states in conditions that eliminate central vision and fixation. There are many practical ways to achieve this, such as asking the patient to wear underwater goggles covered with opaque tape (this achieves complete darkness) or semitransparent tape (which allows light in, but obscures any other visual input).

Part II

Complex Reflex Epilepsies[1,2,65]

Seizures Induced by Thinking and Praxis[49,52,65,147]

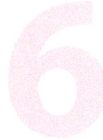

Thinking-induced (noogenic) seizures occur in response to high non-verbal cognitive functions such as mathematical calculations, solving problems, playing games that need mental effort (e.g. chess) and ideation, alone or more often in combination. Praxis-induced seizures are triggered by similar mental activities accompanied by execution of movement (praxis) such as drawing, and playing cards, chess, other board games or with a Rubik's cube. Decision making, spatial tasks, and heightened attention and stress are essential elements in seizure provocation. There is significant overlap between thinking- and praxis-induced seizures and these usually occur in the context of an IGE.[147] They generally start during adolescence and manifest with myoclonic jerks, absences and GTCSs; focal seizures are rare.

C.P. Panayiotopoulos, *Reflex Seizures and Related Epileptic Syndromes*,
DOI 10.1007/978-1-4471-4042-9_6, © Springer-Verlag London 2012

Primary (Idiopathic) Reading Epilepsy

Synonyms: idiopathic reading epilepsy (see author's note below).

Primary (idiopathic) reading epilepsy is a distinctive form of a reflex epilepsy syndrome, which mainly manifests with myoclonic jerks of the masticatory muscles.[37,38,40,41,52]

Reading (the stimulus) is a well-documented provocative, seizure-inducing stimulus in idiopathic (primary reading epilepsy) and less often cryptogenic/symptomatic epilepsies (Fig. 7.1).[37-41,148-151] In some patients with mainly symptomatic causes, reading provokes focal seizures that are relatively longer than those of the primary reading epilepsy and manifest with alexia and possibly dysphasia without jaw myoclonus (Fig. 7.1c).[40]

Author's note: In ILAE terminology, idiopathic has replaced the word primary and this should also apply to idiopathic (primary) reading epilepsy.

Clarifications on Classification

Primary reading epilepsy is classified in the 1989 ILAE classification[4] among the 'idiopathic, age- and localisation-related (partial) epilepsies'. The new ILAE diagnostic scheme (Table 1) now rightly categorises 'reading epilepsy' as a syndrome of reflex epilepsy.[5]

Demographic Data

Onset ranges between 12 and 19 years with a peak in the late teens, which is long after reading skills have been acquired. There is a male preponderance of 1.8/1. The prevalence may be very low (0.2% among patients with onset of non-febrile seizures between birth and 15 years of age).[109]

Clinical Manifestations

Seizures are elicited by reading and consist of brief myoclonic jerks mainly restricted to the masticatory, oral and perioral muscles. They are described as clicking sensations and occur a few minutes to hours after reading. If the patient continues reading despite jaw jerks, these may become more violent, spread to the trunk and limb muscles or generate other seizure manifestations before a GTCS develops. This is usually the first and last GTCS in the patient's life, because the condition is effectively treated and the patient learns to stop

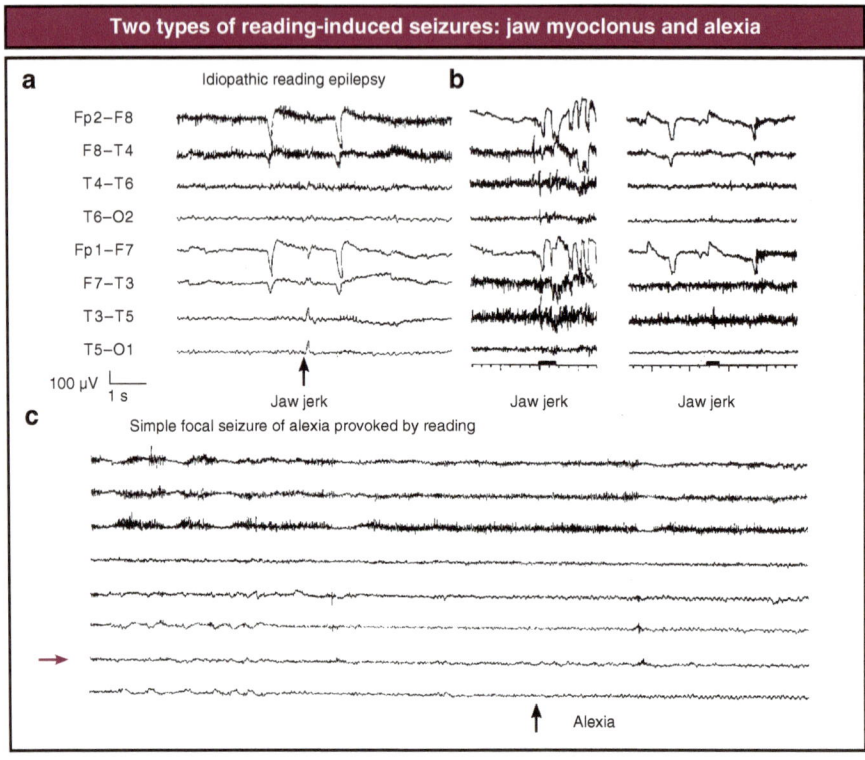

Fig. 7.1 (**a**) The EEG of a woman with jaw jerks (*arrow*) while reading (case 8 in Koutroumanidis et al.[40]). She is successfully treated with clonazepam 0.5 mg at night. Her sister also suffered from jaw jerks, mainly when involved in argumentative and fast talk. (**b**) Video-EEG of another woman with jaw jerks (bars) while reading (case 10 in Koutroumanidis et al.[40]). The EEG shows no detectable abnormality during jaw jerks and possible changes are obscured by muscle activity. (**c**) Video-EEG of a 24-year-old man with simple focal seizures manifested with alexia (inability to understand written words) and four nocturnal GTCSs (case 17 in Koutroumanidis et al.[40]). The inter-ictal EEG during reading showed sharp and slow waves focused in the left posterior temporal regions (*red arrow*). When the patient indicated his inability to understand text (*arrow*), the EEG showed low-amplitude fast rhythms (around 10 or 11 Hz), which were localised in the left posterior temporal regions (*red arrow*). This lasted 70 s before clinical recovery. MRI and a PET scan were normal. The patient was effectively treated with carbamazepine (Modified with permission from Panayiotopoulos[8])

reading or talking when oral/perioral jerks occur. It is extremely rare for patients with reading epilepsy to have more than one to five GTCSs or spontaneous seizures unrelated to reading. Other types of ictal manifestations (mainly visual hallucinations) rarely occur. One of my patients, a 23-year-old woman with primary reading epilepsy, had olfactory hallucinations after repetitive jaw myoclonus induced by prolonged reading or argumentative talking. Occasionally, absences may occur.

Hand myoclonic jerking is common among those with seizures precipitated by writing (*graphogenic epilepsy*).[43]

Precipitating Factors

The stimulus is reading silently or aloud, particularly texts that are difficult to understand or are unusual. Approximately a quarter of patients may also have similar jaw jerks that are provoked by talking (particularly if this is fast or argumentative), writing, reading music or chewing. Clinically identical seizures can also be provoked by other linguistic activities, thus justifying the term 'language-induced epilepsy'.[40,43]

Aetiology

Idiopathic reading epilepsy is probably genetically determined and has been reported in identical twins and among first-degree relatives.[37]

Focal epileptic seizures provoked by reading that manifest with alexia without jaw jerks and last for minutes are probably of cryptogenic or symptomatic cause (Fig. 7.1c).[40]

Pathophysiology

Ictogenesis in reading or language-induced epilepsy is attributed to reflex activation of a hyperexcitable network that subserves the function of speech and extends over multiple cerebral areas on both hemispheres. The parts of this network responding to the stimulus may drive the relative motor areas producing the typical regional myoclonus.[40] The main mechanism is attributed to the transformation, transcoding written linguistic symbols into phonematic, loud or silent speech.[37,150] This may be enhanced by other superimposed factors, such as proprioceptive impulses from oral, perioral and eye muscles involved in reading, and difficulty in transcoding script into speech.[37]

Brain opioid-like substances may be involved in the termination of reading-induced seizures.[148]

Diagnostic Procedures

All tests apart from the EEG are normal. In symptomatic and cryptogenic forms, brain MRI may show abnormalities in the dominant posterior temporal area.[40]

An unusual gyrus branching anteriorly off the left central sulcus has been shown with fMRI.[151]

Electroencephalography[40]

The inter-ictal EEG is usually normal.

Ictal EEG manifestations are often inconspicuous because of jaw muscle artefacts. Ictal EEG changes are variable in terms of morphology and topography. Commonly, they consist of bilateral sharp waves in the temporoparietal regions with left-sided emphasis (Fig. 7.1). Ictal discharges of alexia (symptomatic seizures) are prolonged and entirely focal in the language-dominant temporoparietal regions.

Prognosis

The prognosis of idiopathic reading epilepsy is good, because seizures are usually mild and related to a precipitating stimulus that can be modified.

Management

Modification of reading and talking habits may be successful.

Clonazepam 0.5–1.0 mg at night is highly effective. Some authors use valproate but this may not be needed for the majority of patients who do extremely well on clonazepam alone.

Focal seizures with alexia as a main manifestation do not usually respond to clonazepam or valproate and may also be resistant to carbamazepine.

Startle Seizures

Synonym: startle-induced seizures, startle epilepsy.

Startle seizures are induced by sudden and unexpected stimuli.[56,152-158] The startle (unexpected and sudden presentation of the stimulus) is the provoking factor, although, rarely, patients may be specifically sensitive to one sensory modality. Sudden noise is the main triggering stimulus, but somatosensory and, less often, visual stimuli also effectively trigger seizures in some patients. Habituation to repetitive stimulation occurs.

Clarifications on Classification

The 1989 ILAE definition for startle seizures is:

> *Epileptic seizures may also be precipitated by sudden arousal (startle epilepsy); the stimulus is unexpected in nature. The seizures are usually generalized tonic but may be partial and are usually symptomatic.*[4]

The ILAE diagnostic scheme considered 'startle epilepsy' to be a syndrome, although most realistically this is a type of startle-induced seizure that occurs in a heterogeneous group of patients of variable aetiologies and EEG correlates.[157] This, as was suggested in the main edition of my book 83a, has now been corrected in the new ILAE report, which does not include 'startle epilepsy' in the list of proposed epileptic syndromes (Table 1).[6]

Demographic Data

Onset is in childhood or early adolescence (1–16 years). Both sexes are equally affected. The prevalence is very low.

Clinical Manifestations[56,154,157]

Most patients have static neurological and intellectual handicaps. Infantile hemiplegia predominates.

The startle response is brief (up to 30 s) and consists of axial tonic posturing, frequently causing falls, which can often be traumatic. The seizures are asymmetrical in approximately a quarter of patients. In hemiparetic patients, the seizure starts with flexion and abduction of the paretic arm and extension of the ipsilateral leg, and rapidly involves the contralateral side. Concurrent

C.P. Panayiotopoulos, *Reflex Seizures and Related Epileptic Syndromes*, DOI 10.1007/978-1-4471-4042-9_8, © Springer-Verlag London 2012

symptoms, such as marked autonomic manifestations, automatisms, laughter and jerks, may occur.Less commonly, startle-induced seizures may be atonic or myoclonic, particularly in patients with cerebral anoxia. Seizures are frequent, occurring many times a day, and sometimes progress to status epilepticus.

Spontaneous seizures are common (probably all patients), but infrequent and may precede or follow the startle-induced seizures.

Aetiology

Startle-induced seizures usually occur in patients with a variety of localised or diffuse static brain pathology (*symptomatic startle seizures*). Typically, the insults are pre- or perinatal, or occur within the first 2 years of life. Startle-induced seizures appear to be common in Down syndrome.[159]

Diagnostic Procedures

A variety of focal and diffuse, usually atrophic and often large, cerebral abnormalities are found. Brain MRI is necessary even in those patients with normal neurology.[154] The abnormalities are found predominantly in the lateral sensorimotor cortex.

Electroencephalography

The inter-ictal EEG shows a variety of diffuse or focal abnormalities reflecting the underlying brain structural lesions.

The ictal EEG consists of an initial vertex discharge followed by diffuse relative flattening or low-voltage rhythmic activity of about 10 Hz, which begins in the lesioned motor or premotor cortex, and spreads to mesial frontal, parietal and contralateral frontal regions.[152,154,155] On the surface EEG, this is often obscured by muscle artefacts.

Differential Diagnosis

The main diagnostic confusion is with hyperekplexia (also called startle disease), which is a non-epileptic disorder.

Seizures induced by touch, tap or sudden dousing with hot water may have a startle component, but this is not a prerequisite for their provocation. In addition, these reflex seizures are mainly myoclonic, the ictal EEG shows generalised discharges, patients are otherwise normal and there are no structural brain abnormalities.

Prognosis

The prognosis is often poor, particularly for those with severe pre-existing encephalopathies. The mortality rate is increased compared with that of the general population. Total control of the seizures is almost impossible.

Management

There is no established drug of choice, and therapy is often unsatisfactory. Clonazepam, clobazam and carbamazepine are frequently used. The role of the newer AEDs in startle seizures has not been investigated. Lamotrigine[160] and levetiracetam[161] have been found to be very effective in small series of patients.

Hot Water Epilepsy

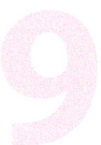

Synonyms: water immersion epilepsy, bathing epilepsy.

Hot water epilepsy is a term used to encompass a reflex epileptic condition characterised by epileptic seizures elicited by pouring hot water (40–50°C) over the head.[24,162-170] Thus, this mode of reflex epilepsy requires a specific thermal cutaneous (i.e. pouring of very hot water over the head) stimulus.

Less often, seizures may occur while using a shower, during tub bathing or exceptionally with cold water.[171] A particular type of soap and entry of water into the mouth are unusual triggering factors.

At a later stage in the natural history, 5–10% of these patients have seizures during a bath even when water is not poured over the head.[170]

Self-induction occurs in 10–20% of patients.[169,171]

Clarifications on Classification

The ILAE Task Force core group has introduced 'hot water epilepsy in infants' as a new reflex epileptic syndrome with a relative confidence level of 2 (Table 1).[6]

Author's note: I do not endorse 'in infants' as part of the nomenclature of this syndrome because of its wide age range at onset.

Demographic Data

Age at onset of the first reflex seizure is from 2 months to 58 years with a mean of 13 years.[24,168,170]

Half of patients have their first seizure during the first decade of life but in a third, this happens after the age of 18 years. Male patients outnumber females in a ratio of 3:1. Boys are two- to three times more frequently affected than girls. The prevalence is very low.

Hot water epilepsy has been mainly described in India and Turkey but case reports have been published from many other countries.

In India, estimated incidence is 60 per 100,000 in Bangalore and 255 per 100,000 in Yelandur.[163,170] This high incidence may be due to a racially determined genetic trait, bathing habits or both.

C.P. Panayiotopoulos, *Reflex Seizures and Related Epileptic Syndromes*, DOI 10.1007/978-1-4471-4042-9_9, © Springer-Verlag London 2012

Clinical Manifestations

Hot water-induced seizures are predominantly (80%) simple or complex focal with (25%) or without (75%) secondarily GTCSs.[24,163,168,170]

Onsets are described as staring, incomprehensible speech, déjà vu, fainting-like sensations, tinnitus, nausea, vomiting, confusion, feeling of pleasure or fear, relaxation or calmness, visual, auditory, olfactory (taste of soap) halluci-nations and complex automatisms.

Primarily GTCSs are reported much less often and certainly not more than in a fourth of patients.

The seizures may occur at any time during the bathing, even at the begin-ning of it. Their duration is usually 30 s to 3 min.

Generally, the frequency of these seizures depends on the frequency of head bathing.[170]

One fourth to a half of patients also have spontaneous seizures (some of them are nocturnal GTCSs), which begin within 1–6 years after the onset of the reflex seizures.[24,168,170] One such patient had IPOS.[24]

Self-induced seizures: 10–20% of patients experience intense pleasure (sometimes described as sexual pleasure) during the seizures.[24,170,172] They self-induce seizures by increasing the temperature of the water and pouring more hot water over their head until they lose consciousness. Self-induction mainly occurs towards the end of the bath. Contrary to other patients with self-induced seizures, such as in photosensitive epilepsy, these patients are not embarrassed talking about their self-induced experiences (including feelings of arousal)[24] and details of the methods of self-induction.

Aetiology

Almost all cases of hot water epilepsy are seen in otherwise healthy children with normal neurological examination and normal brain imaging.

Febrile seizures do not appear to be higher among these patients. However, almost half of them have other family members with various but non-defined types of epilepsy. Familial cases with more than one member having hot water epilepsy have been reported in 18% of the patients from India[170] and in 10% from Turkey.[168] Because of the high frequency of consanguineous marriages in these countries, autosomal recessive inheritance is likely.[169]

In a recent study[169] of a large four-generation family with autosomal domi-nant inheritance of hot water epilepsy, significant linkage was detected on chromosome 4q24-q28, with the highest two-point LOD score of 3.50 at recombination value (theta) of 0 for the marker D4S402. The critical genetic interval spans 22.5 cM and corresponds to about 24 megabases of DNA. Suggested candidate genes for hot water epilepsy include *NEUROG2, ANK2, UGT8* and *CAMK2D*.[169]

Pathophysiology

In a recent experimental study, kindling was demonstrated in association with hyperthermic seizures induced by repeated hot water stimulation in a male Wistar albino rat model.[173] Following 8–12 episodes of hot water stimulations there was progressive epileptic activity[173] manifested in the form of:

- A lowering of rectal temperature thresholds from 41.5°C to 40.0°C
- A drop in latency for developing seizures from 185 to 118 s
- An increase in duration of hippocampal seizure discharge from 15 to 140 s
- A progressive increase in complexity of EEG after discharges
- An increase in behavioural seizure severity from Grade 1 to 5 in all the rats
- Neuronal sprouting observed in the supragranular molecular layer and stratum lacunosum

Diagnostic Procedures

Brain imaging is usually normal, although abnormalities have been described in a few cases.[174] One patient out of 25 had MRI findings consistent with hippocampal sclerosis.[24]

Electroencephalography[24,168,170]

The inter-ictal EEG may be normal for half of the patients. The others show mainly unilateral temporal lobe abnormalities of spikes, sharp waves or slow waves only.

The ictal EEG starts with focal, usually unilateral, rhythmic slow-wave activity of high amplitude, often intermixed with spikes.[170,175]

Differential Diagnosis

The differential diagnosis includes heat-induced vagal syncopes, febrile seizures and breath-holding syncopal attacks.

Prognosis

Hot water epilepsy usually has a good prognosis and is self-limited.

Management

Altering the bathing techniques, by lowering water temperature, showering or sponging instead of pouring water over the head, and reducing the duration of the bath are usually sufficient to achieve seizure control. AEDs are only indicated when these stimulus-modifying or -preventing measures fail or when spontaneous seizures also occur. Intermittent oral administration of clobazam before a hot water bath has been found to be effective.[176] Withdrawal of medication should start upon remission of seizures.

References

1. Beaumanoir A, Gastaut H, Roger J, editors. Reflex seizures and reflex epilepsies. Geneve: Medecine and Hygiene; 1989.
2. Zifkin B, Andermann F, Rowan AJ, Beaumanoir A, editors. Reflex epilepsies and reflex seizures. Advances in neurology, vol 75. New York: Lippincot-Raven; 1998.
3. Wolf P, Inoue Y, Zifkin B, editors. Reflex epilepsies: progress in understanding. Montrouge: John Libbey Eurotext; 2004.
4. Commission on Classification and Terminology of the International League Against Epilepsy. Proposal for revised classification of epilepsies and epileptic syndromes. Epilepsia. 1989;30:389–99.
5. Engel Jr J. A proposed diagnostic scheme for people with epileptic seizures and with epilepsy: report of the ILAE Task Force on Classification and Terminology. Epilepsia. 2001;42:796–803.
6. Engel Jr J. Report of the ILAE Classification Core Group. Epilepsia. 2006;47:1558–68.
7. Blume WT, Luders HO, Mizrahi E, Tassinari C, van Emde BW, Engel Jr J. Glossary of descriptive terminology for ictal semiology: report of the ILAE task force on classification and terminology. Epilepsia. 2001;42:1212–8.
8. Panayiotopoulos CP. Epilepsies characterized by seizures with specific modes of precipitation (reflex epilepsies). In: Wallace S, editor. Epilepsy in children. London: Chapman & Hall; 1996. p. 355–75.
9. Duncan JS, Panayiotopoulos CP. Typical absences with specific modes of precipitation (reflex absences): clinical aspects. In: Duncan JS, Panayiotopoulos CP, editors. Typical absences and related epileptic syndromes. London: Churchill Communications Europe; 1995. p. 206–12.
10. Ferrie CD, De Marco P, Grunewald RA, Giannakodimos S, Panayiotopoulos CP. Video game induced seizures. J Neurol Neurosurg Psychiatry. 1994;57:925–31.
11. Ferrie CD, Robinson RO, Giannakodimos S, Panayiotopoulos CP. Video-game epilepsy. Lancet. 1994; 344:1710–1.
12. Panayiotopoulos CP. Benign childhood partial seizures and related epileptic syndromes. London: John Libbey & Co. Ltd; 1999.
13. Harding GFA, Jeavons PM. Photosensitive epilepsy. London: MacKeith Press; 1994.
14. Wilkins A. Visual stress. Oxford University Press: Oxford; 1995.
15. Zifkin BG, Kasteleijn-Nolst TD. Reflex epilepsy and reflex seizures of the visual system: a clinical review. Epileptic Disord. 2000;2:129–36.
16. Takahashi T. Photosensitive epilepsy. EEG diagnosis by low-luminance, visual stimuli and preventive measures. Tokyo: Igaku-Shoin Publication Service Ltd.; 2002.
17. Forster FM, Cleeland CS. Somatosensory evoked epilepsy. Trans Am Neurol Assoc. 1969;94:268–9.
18. DeMarco P. Parietal epilepsy with evoked and spontaneous spikes: report on siblings with possible genetic transmission. Clin Electroencephalogr. 1986;17:159–61.
19. Fonseca LC, Tedrus GM. Somatosensory evoked spikes and epileptic seizures: a study of 385 cases. Clin Electroencephalogr. 2000;31:71–5.
20. Tedrus GM, Fonseca LC. Benign focal epilepsy of childhood: epileptic seizure during somatosensory evoked potential: a case report. Clin EEG Neurosci. 2004;35:94–6.
21. Deonna T. Reflex seizures with somatosensory precipitation. Clinical and electroencephalographic patterns and differential diagnosis, with emphasis on reflex myoclonic epilepsy of infancy. Adv Neurol. 1998; 75:193–206.
22. Koutroumanidis M, Pearce R, Sadoh DR, Panayiotopoulos CP. Tooth brushing-induced seizures: a case report. Epilepsia. 2001;42:686–8.
23. Chuang YC, Lin TK, Lui CC, Chen SD, Chang CS. Tooth-brushing epilepsy with ictal orgasms. Seizure. 2004; 13:179–82.
24. Yalcin AD, Toydemir HE, Forta H. Hot water epilepsy: clinical and electroencephalographic features of 25 cases. Epilepsy Behav. 2006;9:89–94.
25. Dreifuss FE. Classification of reflex epilepsies and reflex seizures. Adv Neurol. 1998;75:5–13.
26. Duncan JS, Panayiotopoulos CP. The differentiation of 'eye-closure' from 'eye-closed' EEG abnormalities and their relation to photo- and fixation-off sensitivity. In: Duncan JS, Panayiotopoulos CP, editors. Eyelid myoclonia with absences. London: John Libbey & Co. Ltd; 1996. p. 77–87.

27. Beaumanoir A, Mira L, van Lierde A. Epilepsy or paroxysmal kinesigenic choreoathetosis? Brain Dev. 1996;18:139–41.
28. Spinnler H. Valli G [Micturition "reflex" epilepsy. Presentation of a clinical case.]. Riv Patol Nerv Ment. 1969;90:212–20.
29. Rathore C, Radhakrishnan A, Nayak SD, Radhakrishnan K. Teaching video neuroimage: electroclinical characteristics of micturition-induced reflex epilepsy. Neurology. 2008;70:e86.
30. Senanayake N. 'Eating epilepsy' – a reappraisal. Epilepsy Res. 1990;5:74–9.
31. Remillard GM, Zifkin BG, Andermann F. Seizures induced by eating. Adv Neurol. 1998;75:227–40.
32. Tassinari CA, Rubboli G, Rizzi R, Gardella E, Michelucci R. Self-induction of visually-induced seizures. Adv Neurol. 1998;75:179–92.
33. Binnie CD, Wilkins AJ. Visually induced seizures not caused by flicker (intermittent light stimulation). Adv Neurol. 1998;75:123–38.
34. Radhakrishnan K, Klass DW. Half a century of visual pattern-sensitive epilepsy. Mayo Clin Proc. 2004; 79:269–70.
35. Panayiotopoulos CP. Self-induced pattern-sensitive epilepsy. Arch Neurol. 1979;36:48–50.
36. Panayiotopoulos CP. Fixation-off, scotosensitive, and other visual-related epilepsies. Adv Neurol. 1998; 75:139–57.
37. Wolf P. Reading epilepsy. In: Roger J, Bureau M, Dravet C, Dreifuss FE, Perret A, Wolf P, editors. Epileptic syndromes in infancy, childhood and adolescence. London: John Libbey & Co. Ltd; 1992. p. 281–98.
38. Radhakrishnan K, Silbert PL, Klass DW. Reading epilepsy. An appraisal of 20 patients diagnosed at the Mayo Clinic, Rochester, Minnesota, between 1949 and 1989, and delineation of the epileptic syndrome. Brain. 1995;118(Pt 1):75–89.
39. Koepp MJ, Hansen ML, Pressler RM, Brooks DJ, Brandl U, Guldin B, et al. Comparison of EEG, MRI and PET in reading epilepsy: a case report. Epilepsy Res. 1998;29:251–7.
40. Koutroumanidis M, Koepp MJ, Richardson MP, Camfield C, Agathonikou A, Ried S, et al. The variants of reading epilepsy. A clinical and video-EEG study of 17 patients with reading-induced seizures. Brain. 1998;121(Pt 8):1409–27.
41. Ramani V. Reading epilepsy. Adv Neurol. 1998;75:241–62.
42. Cirignotta F, Zucconi M, Mondini S, Lugaresi E. Writing epilepsy. Clin Electroencephalogr. 1986;17: 21–3.
43. Oshima T, Hirose K, Murakami H, Suzuki S, Kanemoto K. Graphogenic epilepsy: a variant of language-induced epilepsy distinguished from reading- and praxis-induced epilepsy. Seizure. 2003;12:56–9.
44. Wieser HG. Seizure induction in reflex seizures and reflex epilepsy. Adv Neurol. 1998;75:69–85.
45. Martinez-Manas R, Daniel RT, Debatisse D, Maeder-Ingvar M, Meagher-Villemure K, Villemure JG, et al. Intractable reflex audiogenic epilepsy successfully treated by peri-insular hemispherotomy. Seizure. 2004;13:486–90.
46. Wieser HG, Hungerbuhler H, Siegel AM, Buck A. Musicogenic epilepsy: review of the literature and case report with ictal single photon emission computed tomography. Epilepsia. 1997;38:200–7.
47. Pittau F, Tinuper P, Bisulli F, Naldi I, Cortelli P, Bisulli A, et al. Videopolygraphic and functional MRI study of musicogenic epilepsy. A case report and literature review. Epilepsy Behav. 2008;13:685–92.
48. Michelucci R, Gardella E, de Haan GJ, Bisulli F, Zaniboni A, Cantalupo G, et al. Telephone-induced seizures: a new type of reflex epilepsy. Epilepsia. 2004;45:280–3.
49. Inoue Y, Zifkin BG. Praxis induction and thinking induction: one or two mechanisms? A controversy. In: Wolf P, Inoue Y, Zifkin B, editors. Reflex epilepsies: progress in understanding. Montrouge: John Libbey Eurotext; 2004. p. 41–55.
50. Andermann F, Zifkin BG, Andermann E. Epilepsy induced by thinking and spatial tasks. Adv Neurol. 1998;75:263–72.
51. Koutroumanidis M, Agathonikou A, Panayiotopoulos CP. Self induced noogenic seizures in a photosensitive patient. J Neurol Neurosurg Psychiatry. 1998;64:139–40.
52. Wolf P, Inoue Y. Complex reflex epilepsies: reading epilepsy and praxis induction. In: Roger J, Bureau M, Dravet C, Genton P, Tassinari CA, Wolf P, editors. Epileptic syndromes in infancy, childhood and adolescence. 4th ed. Montrouge: John Libbey Eurotext Ltd; 2005. p. 347–58.
53. Rocand JC, Graveleau D, Etienne M, Le Balle JC, Laplane R. [Emotionally precipitated epilepsy. Its relations to hysteroepilepsy and reflex epilepsy. Apropos of a case.]. Ann Pediatr (Paris). 1965;12:434–9.
54. Gras P, Grosmaire N, Giroud M, Soichot P. Dumas R [Investigation via electroencephalogram with sphenoidal electrodes of a case of reading epilepsy: role of the temporal lobe in the emotional evocation of seizures.]. Neurophysiol Clin. 1992;22:313–20.
55. Schondienst M. Emotional seizure precipitation and psychogenic epileptic seizures. In: Wolf P, Inoue Y, Zifkin B, editors. Reflex epilepsies: progress in understanding. Montrouge: John Libbey Eurotext; 2004. p. 93–104.

56. Zifkin B, Andermann F. Startle epilepsy. 2011. http://www.ilae-epilepsy.org/Visitors/Centre/ctf/startle.cfm. Last accessed 10 Sep 2011.

57. Panayiotopoulos CP. The epilepsies: seizures, syndromes and management. Oxford: Bladon Medical Publishing; 2005.

58. Panayiotopoulos CP. A practical guide to childhood epilepsies. The educational kit on epilepsies. Oxford: Medicinae; 2006.

59. Panayiotopoulos CP, editor. Idiopathic generalised epilepsies with myoclonic jerks. Oxford: Medicinae; 2007.

60. Kasteleijn-Nolst Trenite DG, Silva AM, Ricci S, Rubboli G, Tassinari CA, Lopes J, et al. Video games are exciting: a European study of video game-induced seizures and epilepsy. [Published with videosequences.]. Epileptic Disord. 2002;4:121–8.

61. Gastaut H, Regis H, Bostem F. Attacks provoked by television, and their mechanisms. Epilepsia. 1962;3:438–45.

62. Gastaut H, Tassinari CA. Triggering mechanisms in epilepsy. The electroclinical point of view. Epilepsia. 1966;7:85–138.

63. Panayiotopoulos CP, Jeavons PM, Harding GF. Occipital spikes and their relation to visual responses in epilepsy, with particular reference to photosensitive epilepsy. Electroencephalogr Clin Neurophysiol. 1972;32:179–90.

64. Panayiotopoulos CP. A study of photosensitive epilepsy with particular reference to occipital spikes induced by intermittent photic stimulation. Birmingham: Aston University; 1972. p. 1–289.

65. Zifkin BG, Guerrini R, Plouin P. Simple reflex epilepsies. In: Engel Jr J, Pedley TA, editors. Epilepsy: a comprehensive textbook, vol. III. 2nd ed. Philadelphia: Lippincott Williams and Wilkins; 2008. p. 2559–74.

66. Wolf P, Goosses R. Relation of photosensitivity to epileptic syndromes. J Neurol Neurosurg Psychiatry. 1986;49:1386–91.

67. Gowers WR. Epilepsies and other chronic convulsive diseases. Their causes, symptoms and treatment. London: Churchill JA; 1881.

68. Gastaut H, Roger J, Gastaut Y. Les formes experimentales de l' epilepsie humaine: 1. L' epilepsie induite par la stimulation lumineuse intermittente rythmee ou epilepsie photogenique. Rev Neurol (Paris). 1948; 80:161–83.

69. Bickford RG, Daly DD, Keith HM. Convulsive effects of light stimulation in children. Am J Dis Child. 1953;86:170–83.

70. Panayiotopoulos CP, Jeavons PM, Harding GF. Relation of occipital spikes evoked by intermittent photic stimulation to visual evoked responses in photosensitive epilepsy. Nature. 1970;228:566–7.

71. Tassinari CA, Rubboli G, Plasmati R, Salvi F, Ambrosetto G, Bianchedi G, et al. Television-induced epilepsy with occipital seizures. In: Beaumanoir A, Gastaut H, Naquet R, editors. Reflex seizures and reflex epilepsies. Geneva: Editions Medecine & Hygiene; 1989. p. 241–3.

72. Aso K, Watanabe K, Negoro T, Furune A, Takahashi I, Yamamoto N, et al. Photosensitive partial seizure: the origin of abnormal discharges. J Epilepsy. 1988;1:87–93.

73. Guerrini R, Dravet C, Genton P, Bureau M, Bonanni P, Ferrari AR, et al. Idiopathic photosensitive occipital lobe epilepsy. Epilepsia. 1995;36:883–91.

74. Takada H, Aso K, Watanabe K, Okumura A, Negoro T, Ishikawa T. Epileptic seizures induced by animated cartoon, 'Pocket Monster'. Epilepsia. 1999;40:997–1002.

75. Guerrini R, Bonanni P, Parmeggiani L, Thomas P, Mattia D, Harvey AS, et al. Induction of partial seizures by visual stimulation. Clinical and electroencephalographic features and evoked potential studies. Adv Neurol. 1998;75:159–78.

76. De Bittencourt PR. Photosensitivity: the magnitude of the problem. Epilepsia. 2004;45 Suppl 1:30–4.

77. Fisher RS, Harding G, Erba G, Barkley GL, Wilkins A. Photic- and pattern-induced seizures: a review for the Epilepsy Foundation of America Working Group. Epilepsia. 2005;46:1426–41.

78. Quirk JA, Fish DR, Smith SJ, Sander JW, Shorvon SD, Allen PJ. First seizures associated with playing electronic screen games: a community-based study in Great Britain. Ann Neurol. 1995;37:733–7.

79. Quirk JA, Fish DR, Smith SJ, Sander JW, Shorvon SD, Allen PJ. Incidence of photosensitive epilepsy: a prospective national study. Electroencephalogr Clin Neurophysiol. 1995;95:260–7.

80. Grecory RP, Oates T, Merry RTC. EEG epileptiform abnormalities in candidates for aircrew training. Electroencephalogr Clin Neurophysiol. 1993;86:75–7.

81. Kasteleijn-Nolst Trenite DG, Binnie CD, Meinardi H. Photosensitive patients: symptoms and signs during intermittent photic stimulation and their relation to seizures in daily life. J Neurol Neurosurg Psychiatry. 1987;50:1546–9.

82. Kasteleijn-Nolst Trenite DG. Photosensitivity in epilepsy: electrophysiological and clinical correlates. Acta Neurol Scand Suppl. 1989;125:3–149.

83. Benbadis SR, Gerson WA, Harvey JH, Luders HO. Photosensitive temporal lobe epilepsy. Neurology. 1996;46:1540–2.

83a. Panayiotopoulos CP. A clinical guide to epileptic syndromes and their treatment. Revised 2nd edition. London: Springer, 2010

84. Graf WD, Chatrian GE, Glass ST, Knauss TA. Video game-related seizures: a report on 10 patients and a review of the literature. Pediatrics. 1994;93:551–6.

85. Panayiotopoulos CP, Giannakodimos S, Agathonikou A, Koutroumanidis M. Eyelid myoclonia is not a manoeuvre for self-induced seizures in eyelid myoclonia with absences. In: Duncan JS, Panayiotopoulos CP, editors. Eyelid myoclonia with absences. London: John Libbey & Co. Ltd; 1996. p. 93–106.

86. Binnie CD. Differential diagnosis of eyelid myoclonia with absences and self-induction by eye closure. In: Duncan JS, Panayiotopoulos CP, editors. Eyelid myoclonia with absences. London: John Libbey & Co. Ltd; 1996. p. 89–92.

87. Ames FR, Saffer D. The sunflower syndrome. A new look at "self-induced" photosensitive epilepsy. J Neurol Sci. 1983;59:1–11.

88. Stephani U, Tauer U, Koeleman B, Pinto D, Neubauer BA, Lindhout D. Genetics of photosensitivity (photoparoxysmal response): a review. Epilepsia. 2004;45 Suppl 1:19–23.

89. Harding GF, Edson A, Jeavons PM. Persistence of photosensitivity. Epilepsia. 1997;38:663–9.

90. Pinto D, Westland B, de Haan GJ, Rudolf G, da Silva BM, Hirsch E, et al. Genome-wide linkage scan of epilepsy-related photoparoxysmal EEG response: evidence for linkage on chromosomes 7q32 and 16p13. Hum Mol Genet. 2005;14:171–8.

91. Pinto D, Kasteleijn-Nolst Trenite DG, Cordell HJ, Mattheisen M, Strauch K, Lindhout D, et al. Explorative two-locus linkage analysis suggests a multiplicative interaction between the 7q32 and 16p13 myoclonic seizures-related photosensitivity loci. Genet Epidemiol. 2007;31:42–50.

92. Tauer U, Lorenz S, Lenzen KP, Heils A, Muhle H, Gresch M, et al. Genetic dissection of photosensitivity and its relation to idiopathic generalized epilepsy. Ann Neurol. 2005;57:866–73.

93. Dibbens LM, Ekberg J, Taylor I, Hodgson BL, Conroy SJ, Lensink IL, et al. NEDD4-2 as a potential candidate susceptibility gene for epileptic photosensitivity. Genes Brain Behav. 2007;6:750–5.

94. de Haan GJ, Trenite DK, Stroink H, Parra J, Voskuyl R, van Kempen M, et al. Monozygous twin brothers discordant for photosensitive epilepsy: first report of possible visual priming in humans. Epilepsia. 2005;46:1545–9.

95. Kasteleijn-Nolst Trenite DG, Binnie CD, Harding GF, Wilkins A. Photic stimulation: standardization of screening methods. Epilepsia. 1999;40 Suppl 4:75–9.

96. Kasteleijn-Nolst Trenite DG, Binnie CD, Harding GF, Wilkins A, Covanis T, Eeg-Olofsson O, et al. Medical technology assessment photic stimulation – standardization of screening methods. Neurophysiol Clin. 1999;29:318–24.

97. Jeavons PM, Harding GF, Panayiotopoulos CP, Drasdo N. The effect of geometric patterns combined with intermittent photic stimulation in photosensitive epilepsy. Electroencephalogr Clin Neurophysiol. 1972;33:221–4.

98. Kasteleijn-Nolst Trenite DG. Reflex seizures induced by intermittent light stimulation. Adv Neurol. 1998;75:99–121.

99. Agathonikou A, Panayiotopoulos CP, Koutroumanidis M, Rowlinson A. Idiopathic regional occipital epilepsy imitating migraine. J Epilepsy. 1997;10:287–90.

100. Panayiotopoulos CP. Effectiveness of photic stimulation on various eye-states in photosensitive epilepsy. J Neurol Sci. 1974;23:165–73.

101. Giannakodimos S, Panayiotopoulos CP. Eyelid myoclonia with absences in adults: a clinical and video-EEG study. Epilepsia. 1996;37:36–44.

102. Panayiotopoulos CP. Fixation-off-sensitive epilepsy in eyelid myoclonia with absence seizures. Ann Neurol. 1987;22:87–9.

103. Verrotti A, Tocco AM, Salladini C, Latini G, Chiarelli F. Human photosensitivity: from pathophysiology to treatment. Eur J Neurol. 2005;12:828–41.

104. Wilkins AJ, Baker A, Amin D, Smith S, Bradford J, Zaiwalla Z, et al. Treatment of photosensitive epilepsy using coloured glasses. Seizure. 1999;8:444–9.

105. Capovilla G, Gambardella A, Rubboli G, Beccaria F, Montagnini A, Aguglia U, et al. Suppressive efficacy by a commercially available blue lens on PPR in 610 photosensitive epilepsy patients. Epilepsia. 2006; 47:529–33.

106. Covanis A. Photosensitivity in idiopathic generalized epilepsies. Epilepsia. 2005;46 Suppl 9:67–72.

107. Binnie CD, van Emde BW, Kasteleijn-Nolste-Trenite DG, de Korte RA, Meijer JW, Meinardi H, et al. Acute effects of lamotrigine (BW430C) in persons with epilepsy. Epilepsia. 1986;27:248–54.

108. von Rosenstiel P. Brivaracetam (UCB 34714). Neurotherapeutics. 2007;4:84–7.

109. Panayiotopoulos CP. Reflex seizures and reflex epilepsies. In: Panayiotopoulos CP, editor. The epilepsies: seizures, syndromes and management. Oxford: Bladon Medical Publishing; 2005. p. 449–96.

110. Guerrini R, Bonanni P, Parmeggiani L. Idiopathic photosensitive occipital lobe epilepsy. 2011. http://www.ilae-epilepsy.org/Visitors/Centre/ctf/idio_photo_occi_lobe.html. Last accessed 10 Sep 2011.

111. Gastaut H, Zifkin BG. Benign epilepsy of childhood with occipital spike and wave complexes. In: Andermann F, Lugaresi E, editors. Migraine and epilepsy. Boston: Butterworths; 1987. p. 47–81.

112. Ricci S, Vigevano F. Occipital seizures provoked by intermittent light stimulation: ictal and interictal findings. J Clin Neurophysiol. 1993;10:197–209.
113. Taylor I, Marini C, Johnson MR, Turner S, Berkovic SF, Scheffer IE. Juvenile myoclonic epilepsy and idiopathic photosensitive occipital lobe epilepsy: is there overlap? Brain. 2004;127(Pt 8):1878–86.
114. Michelucci R, Tassinari CA. Television-induced occipital seizures. In: Andermann F, Beaumanoir A, Mira L, Roger J, Tassinari CA, editors. Occipital seizures and epilepsies in children. London: John Libbey & Co. Ltd; 1993. p. 141–4.
115. Guerrini R, Bonanni P, Parmeggiani L, Belmonte A. Adolescent onset of idiopathic photosensitive occipital epilepsy after remission of benign rolandic epilepsy. Epilepsia. 1997;38:777–81.
116. Panayiotopoulos CP. Elementary visual hallucinations, blindness, and headache in idiopathic occipital epilepsy: differentiation from migraine. J Neurol Neurosurg Psychiatry. 1999;66:536–40.
117. Hishikawa Y, Yamamoto J, Furuya E, Yamada Y, Miyazaki K. Photosensitive epilepsy: relationships between the visual evoked responses and the epileptiform discharges induced by intermittent photic stimulation. Electroencephalogr Clin Neurophysiol. 1967;23:320–34.
118. Maheshwari MC. The clinical significance of occipital spikes as a sole response to intermittent photic stimulation. Electroencephalogr Clin Neurophysiol. 1975;39:93–5.
119. Holmes G. Sabill memorial oration on focal epilepsy. Lancet. 1927;i:957–62.
120. Guerrini R, Ferrari AR, Battaglia A, Salvadori P, Bonanni P. Occipitotemporal seizures with ictus emeticus induced by intermittent photic stimulation. Neurology. 1994;44:253–9.
121. Sharief M, Howard RO, Panayiotopoulos CP, Koutroumanidis M, Rowlinson S, Sanders S. Occipital photosensitivity with onset of seizures in adulthood: an unrecognised condition of good prognosis. J Neurol Neurosurg Psychiatry. 2000;68:257.
122. Donnet A, Bartolomei F. Migraine with visual aura and photosensitive epileptic seizures. Epilepsia. 1997;38:1032–4.
123. Duncan JS, Panayiotopoulos CP, editors. Eyelid myoclonia with absences. London: John Libbey & Co. Ltd; 1996.
124. Kent L, Blake A, Whitehouse W. Eyelid myoclonia with absences: phenomenology in children. Seizure. 1998;7:193–9.
125. Striano S, Striano P, Nocerino C, Boccella P, Bilo L, Meo R, et al. Eyelid myoclonia with absences: an overlooked epileptic syndrome? Neurophysiol Clin. 2002;32:287–96.
126. Ferrie CD. Eyelid myoclonia with absences. In: Wallace SJ, Farrell K, editors. Epilepsy in children. 2nd ed. London: Edward Arnold Ltd; 2004. p. 195–8.
127. Covanis A. Eyelid myoclonia and absence. Adv Neurol. 2005;95:185–96.
128. Striano S, Capovilla G, Sofia V, Romeo A, Rubboli G, Striano P, et al. Eyelid myoclonia with absences (Jeavons syndrome): a well-defined idiopathic generalized epilepsy syndrome or a spectrum of photosensitive conditions? Epilepsia. 2009;50 Suppl 5:159.
129. Panayiotopoulos CP. Eyelid myoclonia with and without absences. 2011. http://www.ilae-epilepsy.org/Visitors/Centre/ctf/eyelid_myoclonia_w_wo_abs.html. Last accessed 9 Sep 2011.
130. Walsh FB. Clinical neuro-ophthalmology. 2nd ed. Baltimore: The Williams & Wilkins Co.; 1957. p. 186–245.
131. Bianchi A, the Italian LAE Collaborative Group. Study of concordance of symptoms in families with absence epilepsies. In: Duncan JS, Panayiotopoulos CP, editors. Typical absences and related epileptic syndromes. London: Churchill Communications Europe; 1995. p. 328–37.
132. Parker A, Gardiner RM, Panayiotopoulos CP, Agathonikou A, Ferrie CD. Observations on families with eyelid myoclonia with absences. In: Duncan JS, Panayiotopoulos CP, editors. Eyelid myoclonia with absences. London: John Libbey & Co. Ltd; 1996. p. 107–15.
133. Camfield CS, Camfield PR, Sadler M, Rahey S, Farrell K, Chayasirisobbon S, et al. Paroxysmal eyelid movements: a confusing feature of generalized photosensitive epilepsy. Neurology. 2004;63:40–2.
134. Ferrie CD, Agathonikou A, Parker A, Robinson RO, Panayiotopoulos CP. The spectrum of childhood epilepsies with eyelid myoclonia. In: Duncan JS, Panayiotopoulos CP, editors. Eyelid myoclonia with absences. London: John Libbey & Co. Ltd; 1996. p. 39–48.
135. Radovici MMA, Misirliou VL, Gluckman M. Epilepsy reflex provoquee par excitations optiques des rayons solaires. Revue Neurologique 1932;1:1305–1307 [Translated by Koutroumanidis M. Reflex epilepsy provoked by optic excitation by (means of) sunrays)]. In: Duncan JS, Panayiotopoulos CP, editors. Eyelid myoclonia with absences. London: John Libbey & Co. Ltd; 1996. p. 103–5.
136. Wilkins A. Towards an understanding of reflex epilepsy and absence. In: Duncan JS, Panayiotopoulos CP, editors. Typical absences and related epileptic syndromes. London: Churchill Communications Europe; 1995. p. 196–205.
137. Harding G, Wilkins AJ, Erba G, Barkley GL, Fisher RS. Photic- and pattern-induced seizures: expert consensus of the Epilepsy Foundation of America Working Group. Epilepsia. 2005;46:1423–5.
138. Radhakrishnan K, St Louis EK, Johnson JA, McClelland RL, Westmoreland BF, Klass DW. Pattern-sensitive epilepsy: electroclinical characteristics, natural history, and delineation of the epileptic syndrome. Epilepsia. 2005;46:48–58.

139. Matricardi M, Brinciotti M, Trasatti G, Porro G. Self-induced pattern-sensitive epilepsy in childhood. Acta Paediatr Scand. 1990;79:237–40.
140. Wilkins AJ, Darby CE, Binnie CD. Neurophysiological aspects of pattern-sensitive epilepsy. Brain. 1979; 102:1–25.
141. Agathonikou A, Koutroumanidis M, Panayiotopoulos CP. Fixation-off-sensitive epilepsy with absences and absence status: video-EEG documentation. Neurology. 1997;48:231–4.
142. Agathonikou A, Koutroumanidis M, Panayiotopoulos CP. Fixation-off (Scoto) sensitivity combined with photosensitivity. Epilepsia. 1998;39:552–5.
143. Krakow K, Baxendale SA, Maguire EA, Krishnamoorthy ES, Lemieux L, Scott CA, et al. Fixation-off sensitivity as a model of continuous epileptiform discharges: electroencephalographic, neuropsychological and functional MRI findings. Epilepsy Res. 2000;42:1–6.
144. Iannetti GD, Di Bonaventura C, Pantano P, Giallonardo AT, Romanelli PL, Bozzao L, et al. fMRI/EEG in paroxysmal activity elicited by elimination of central vision and fixation. Neurology. 2002;58:976–9.
145. Kumada S, Kubota M, Hayashi M, Uchiyama A, Kurata K, Kagamihara Y. Fixation-sensitive myoclonus in Lafora disease. Neurology. 2006;66:1574–6.
146. Beaumanoir A, Capizzi G, Nahory A, Yousfi Y. Scotogenic seizures. In: Beaumanoir A, Gastaut H, Roger J, editors. Reflex seizures and reflex epilepsies. Geneve: Medecine and Hygiene; 1989. p. 219–3.
147. Ferlazzo E, Zifkin BG, Andermann E, Andermann F. Cortical triggers in generalized reflex seizures and epilepsies. Brain. 2005;128(Pt 4):700–10.
148. Koepp MJ, Richardson MP, Brooks DJ, Duncan JS. Focal cortical release of endogenous opioids during reading-induced seizures. Lancet. 1998;352:952–5.
149. Mayer T, Wolf P. Reading epilepsy: clinical and genetic background. In: Berkovic SF, Genton P, Hirsch E, Picard F, editors. Genetics of focal epilepsies. London: John Libbey & Co. Ltd; 1999. p. 159–68.
150. Pegna AJ, Picard F, Martory MD, Vuilleumier P, Seeck M, Jallon P, et al. Semantically-triggered reading epilepsy: an experimental case study. Cortex. 1999;35:101–11.
151. Archer JS, Briellmann RS, Syngeniotis A, Abbott DF, Jackson GD. Spike-triggered fMRI in reading epilepsy: involvement of left frontal cortex working memory area. Neurology. 2003;60:415–21.
152. Garcia-Morales I, Maestu F, Perez-Jimenez MA, et al. A clinical and magnetoencephalography study of MRI-negative startle epilepsy. Epilepsy Behav. 2009;16:166–71.
153. Wilkins DE, Hallett M, Wess MM. Audiogenic startle reflex of man and its relationship to startle syndromes. A review. Brain. 1986;109(Pt 3):561–73.
154. Manford MR, Fish DR, Shorvon SD. Startle provoked epileptic seizures: features in 19 patients. J Neurol Neurosurg Psychiatry. 1996;61:151–6.
155. Vignal JP, Biraben A, Chauvel PY, Reutens DC. Reflex partial seizures of sensorimotor cortex (including cortical reflex myoclonus and startle epilepsy). Adv Neurol. 1998;75:207–26.
156. Nolan MA, Otsubo H, Iida K, Minassian BA. Startle-induced seizures associated with infantile hemiplegia: implication of the supplementary motor area. Epileptic Disord. 2005;7:49–52.
157. Tibussek D, Wohlrab G, Boltshauser E, Schmitt B. Proven startle-provoked epileptic seizures in childhood: semiologic and electrophysiologic variability. Epilepsia. 2006;47:1050–8.
158. Bakker MJ, van Dijk JG, van den Maagdenberg AM, Tijssen MA. Startle syndromes. Lancet Neurol. 2006;5:513–24.
159. Guerrini R, Genton P, Bureau M, Dravet C, Roger J. Reflex seizures are frequent in patients with Down syndrome and epilepsy. Epilepsia. 1990;31:406–17.
160. Faught E. Lamotrigine for startle-induced seizures. Seizure. 1999;8:361–3.
161. Gurses C, Alpay K, Ciftci FD, Bebek N, Baykan B, Gokyigit A. The efficacy and tolerability of Levetiracetam as an add-on therapy in patients with startle epilepsy. Seizure. 2008;17:625–30.
162. Stensman R, Ursing B. Epilepsy precipitated by hot water immersion. Neurology. 1971;21:559–62.
163. Mani KS, Mani AJ, Ramesh CK. Hot-water epilepsy – a peculiar type of reflex epilepsy: clinical and EEG features in 108 cases. Trans Am Neurol Assoc. 1974;99:224–6.
164. Gururaj G, Satishchandra P. Correlates of hot water epilepsy in rural south India: a descriptive study. Neuroepidemiology. 1992;11:173–9.
165. Fukuda M, Morimoto T, Nagao H, Kida K. Clinical study of epilepsy with severe febrile seizures and seizures induced by hot water bath. Brain Dev. 1997;19:212–6.
166. Satishchandra P, Ullal GR, Shankar SK. Hot water epilepsy. Adv Neurol. 1998;75:283–93.
167. Ioos C, Fohlen M, Villeneuve N, Badinand-Hubert N, Jalin C, Cheliout-Heraut F, et al. Hot water epilepsy: a benign and unrecognized form. J Child Neurol. 2000;15:125–8.
168. Bebek N, Gurses C, Gokyigit A, Baykan B, Ozkara C, Dervent A. Hot water epilepsy: clinical and electrophysiologic findings based on 21 cases. Epilepsia. 2001;42:1180–4.
169. Ratnapriya R, Satishchandra P, Kumar SD, Gadre G, Reddy R, Anand A. A locus for autosomal dominant reflex epilepsy precipitated by hot water maps at chromosome 10q21.3-q22.3. Hum Genet. 2009; 125:541–9.
170. Satishchandra P. Hot-water epilepsy. Epilepsia. 2003;44 Suppl 1:29–32.

171. Auvin S, Lamblin MD, Pandit F, Bastos M, Derambure P, Vallee L. Hot water epilepsy occurring at temperature below the core temperature. Brain Dev. 2006;28:265–8.
172. Bebek N, Baykan B, Gurses C, Emir O, Gokyigit A. Self-induction behavior in patients with photosensitive and hot water epilepsy: a comparative study from a tertiary epilepsy center in Turkey. Epilepsy Behav. 2006;9:317–26.
173. Ullal GR, Satishchandra P, Kalladka D, Rajashekar K, Archana K, Mahadevan A, et al. Kindling & Mossy fibre sprouting in the rat hippocampus following hot water induced hyperthermic seizures. Indian J Med Res. 2006;124:331–42.
174. Tezer FI, Ertas N, Yalcin D, Saygi S. Hot water epilepsy with cerebral lesion: a report of five cases with cranial MRI findings. Epilepsy Behav. 2006;8:672–6.
175. De KK, Corthouts I, Van CR, Verhelst H. Hot-water epilepsy: a new Caucasian case. Eur J Pediatr. 2005;164:184–5.
176. Dhanaraj M, Jayavelu A. Prophylactic use of clobazam in hot water epilepsy. J Assoc Physicians India. 2003;51:43–4.

Index

A

Absence(s) (absence seizures; petit mal),
    intermittent photic stimulation-
    induced, 24
Alexia, reading epilepsy, 40

B

Bathing epilepsy, 47–49
Brivaracetam (UCB-34714) for
    photosensitive epilepsy, 14

C

Chromosome(s) disorders/abnormalities
    hot water epilepsy, 48
    photosensitive seizures, 8
Clonazepam for photosensitive
    epilepsy, 14
Complex reflex seizures/epilepsy, 37–49
Cryptogenic (probably symptomatic)
    generalised epilepsy/epilepsy
    syndromes and fixation-off
    sensitivity, 31

E

Electroencephalogram (EEG)
    hot water epilepsy, 49
    idiopathic photosensitive occipital
        lobe epilepsy, 17
    Jeavons syndrome, 12, 22, 23
    pattern-sensitive epilepsy, 28, 29
    reading epilepsy, 40, 41
    startle epilepsy, 43
Environmental (external/extrinsic)
    stimuli in pattern-sensitive
    patients, 28–29
Epilepsy syndromes, reflex seizures in,
    3–14

Eye(s)

closed (state of)
    eye-closure vs., 10–13
    Jeavon's syndrome, 12
closure
    eyes closed vs., 10–13
    Jeavon's syndrome, 12, 21–24
    oculomotor symptoms (incl. deviation)
        of Jeavon's syndrome, 12
    open (state of), 10–12
Eyelid movements
    occipital lobe epilepsy, idiopathic
        photosensitive, 18
    photosensitive seizures, 4, 8, 12, 18
Eyelid myoclonia, 21, 22
    with absences (see Jeavons
        syndrome)diagnosis and
        differential diagnosis, 24–25
    in fixation-off sensitivity, 31, 32
    without absences, 22
Eyelid myoclonic status
    epilepticus, 23

F

Fixation-off sensitivity (FOS), 31–34
Focal (partial/local) epilepsy/seizures,
    photically-induced, 7
FOS. See Fixation-off sensitivity (FOS)
Functional neuroimaging in fixation-off
    sensitivity, 33

G

Generalised (bilateral) epilepsy/seizures
    idiopathic (IGE), fixation-off
        sensitivity (FOS) and, 31–34
    reflex
        Jeavons syndrome, 25
        photosensitive seizures, 4–6, 17

C.P. Panayiotopoulos, *Reflex Seizures and Related Epileptic Syndromes*,   59
DOI 10.1007/978-1-4471-4042-9, © Springer-Verlag London 2012

Generalised spike or polyspike–wave
    discharges (GSWDs), 9–11
  in idiopathic photosensitive occipital
    lobe epilepsy, 17
  Jeavons syndrome, 22, 23
Genetics
  Jeavons syndrome, 24
  pattern-senitive epilepsy, 29
  reading epilepsy, 41

H

Hand myoclonic jerks, 40
Hot water epilepsy, 47–49

I

Ictal events (incl. symptoms) of
    idiopathic photosensitive occipital
    lobe epilepsy, 16
Immersion epilepsy, 47–49
Infancy, hot water epilepsy (ILAE
    category) in, 47
Inter-ictal and background EEG
  hot water epilepsy, 49
  startle seizures, 44
Intermittent photic stimulation/IPS (and
    concomitant EEG recording), 3
  absence seizures induced by, 27
  Jeavon's syndrome, 22, 23
  photosensitive epilepsy, 8–9
    idiopathic occipital lobe, 15–20
International League Against Epilepsy
    (ILAE) diagnostic and
    classification scheme
  Jeavon's syndrome not recognised yet,
    21
  occipital lobe epilepsy, idiopathic
    photosensitive, 15
  reflex seizures and epilepsy
    hot water epilepsy in infants, 47
    photosensitivity, 15
    reading epilepsy, 39
    startle seizures, 43

J

Jaw myoclonus, reading epilepsy, 40

Jeavons syndrome (eyelid myoclonia
    with absences), 21–26
  aetiopathophysiology, 24
  classification, 21
  clinical manifestations, 21–23
  demographic data, 21
  diagnostic procedures, 22, 24
    EEG, 12, 21, 22, 24
  differential diagnosis, 24–25
  management, 25–26
  prognosis, 25

L

Lamotrigine
  Jeavons syndrome, 26
  photosensitive epilepsy, 14
Levetiracetam
  Jeavons syndrome, 26
  photosensitive epilepsy, 14

M

Magnetic resonance imaging in fixation-
    off sensitivity, 33
Magnetoencephalography (MEG) in
    fixation-off sensitivity, 33
Migraine, differential diagnosis of visual
    seizures of, 18–19
Movement execution (=praxis), seizures
    induced by, 37
Myoclonus (incl. myoclonic jerks and
    attacks) in reading epilepsy, 39, 40

N

Neuroimaging (brain imaging) in
    fixation-off sensitivity, 33
Noogenic (thinking) epilepsy, 37

O

Occipital (lobe) epilepsy/seizures (OPS)
  idiopathic, 15
    photically-induced, 15–20
  photosensitive/photically-induced,
    3, 7
    idiopathic, 15–20

Occipital (lobe) paroxysms and
    fixation-off sensitivity, 31
Occipital (lobe) spikes, photically-
    induced, 3, 9, 11
    idiopathic photosensitive occipital lobe
        epilepsy, 15, 17, 18, 19

P

Pattern-sensitive epilepsy, 27–29
Photic stimulation, avoidance of
    prolonged, 9
Photoparoxysmal response (PPR;
    paroxysmal activation by photic
    stimulation), 3, 5, 11, 13
    examples, 10
    in idiopathic photosensitive occipital
        lobe epilepsy, 17
Photosensitivity (and photosensitive
    seizures/epilepsy), 3–14
    aetiopathophysiology, 8
    classification, 3
    clinical manifestations, 4–6
    demographic data, 4
    diagnostic procedures, 8–13
    fixation-off sensitivity and, 32
        differentiation, 31, 32
    management, 13–14
    pattern-sensitive epilepsy and,
        relationship between, 27
Posterior spike/polyspike-waves,
    photically-induced, 11
Post-ictal period of idiopathic
    photosensitive occipital lobe
    epilepsy, 16–17
Praxis-induced seizures, 37
Precipitating factors/stimuli (triggers)
    pattern-sensitive epilepsy, 29
    photosensitive epilepsies, 7–8
        avoidance or prevention,
            13, 20
        idiopathic photosensitive occipital
            lobe epilepsy, 17
    reflex seizures/epilepsy
        Jeavons syndrome, 23
        photosensitive epilepsies (*see*
            subheading above)
        reading epilepsy, 41

Prophylaxis/prevention of provocative
    stimuli in photosensitive epilepsy,
    13, 20

R

Reflex seizures/epilepsy, 1–49
    EEG (*see* Electroencephalogram
        (EEG))
Reflex seizures/epilepsy, complex, 36–49

S

Scotosensitive epilepsy, 33
Seizures (fits; convulsions)
    epileptic/afebrile
        in hot water epilepsy, 47–48
        in Jeavon's syndrome, 21–23
        in reading epilepsy, 39–40
        occipital lobe epilepsy, idiopathic
            photosensitive, 16
Self-induced seizures
    eyelid myoclonia and Jeavons
        syndrome, and, 23
    hot water immersion, 48
    pattern-sensitive epilepsy, 27
    photic reflex seizures, 8
Spike/polyspike-waves, 9–11
    idiopathic photosensitive occipital lobe
        epilepsy, 17
    Jeavons syndrome, 22, 24
Startle seizures/epilepsy, 43–45

T

Television epilepsy, 7–8
    avoidance/prevention, 13
Temporoparieto-occipital with occipital
    emphasis spike/polyspike-waves,
    photically-induced, 11
Thinking/thoughts, seizures induced
    by, 37
Tonic-clonic seizures, generalised
    (GTCSs; bilateral tonic-clonic
    seizures; grand mal)
    in Jeavons syndrome, 23
    in reflex seizures
        photosensitive epilepsy, 4
        reading epilepsy, 39, 40

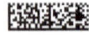

V

Valproate
  photosensitive epilepsy, 14
    idiopathic photosensitive occipital
    lobe epilepsy, 20
  reading epilepsy, 42
Video-game induced seizures, 7
  prevention/avoidance, 13
Visual evoked response/potential (VER;
    VEP)
  photosensitive epilepsy, 11
    idiopathic photosensitive occipital
    lobe epilepsy, 17

Visual seizures and their symptoms (incl.
    hallucinations and illusions)
  differential diagnosis of migraine,
    18–19
  occipital lobe epilepsy, idiopathic
    photosensitive, 16
Visual stimuli (epilepsy precipitated by),
    1–26 *See also* Photosensitivity

W

Writing epilepsy, 40